Fluorinated Carbohydrates

547.781 F673ℓ

ACS SYMPOSIUM SERIES **374**

Fluorinated Carbohydrates

Chemical and Biochemical Aspects

N. F. Taylor, EDITOR

University of Windsor

Developed from a symposium sponsored by
the Division of Carbohydrate Chemistry
at the 194th Meeting
of the American Chemical Society,
New Orleans, Louisiana
August 30–September 4, 1987

American Chemical Society, Washington, DC 1988

Library of Congress Cataloging-in-Publication Data

Fluorinated carbohydrates: chemical and biochemical aspects
  N.F. Taylor, editor

  p.   cm.(ACS Symposium Series: 374).

  Developed from a symposium sponsored by the Division
of Carbohydrate Chemistry at the 194th Meeting of the
American Chemical Society, New Orleans, Louisiana,
August 20–September 4, 1987.
  Includes bibliographies and indexes.

  ISBN 0–8412–1492–1
  1. Fluorocarbohydrates—Physiological effect—
Congresses. 2. Fluorocarbohydrates—Therapeutic use—
Testing—Congresses. 3. Fluorocarbohydrates—
Synthesis—Congresses.

  I. Taylor, N. F. II. American Chemical Society.
Division of Carbohydrate Chemistry. III. Series.

QP702.F58F58   1988
547.7′.81—dc19   88–19332
                                             CIP

ACS Symposium Series

M. Joan Comstock, *Series Editor*

1988 ACS Books Advisory Board

Foreword

The ACS SYMPOSIUM SERIES was founded in 1974 to provide a medium for publishing symposia quickly in book form. The format of the Series parallels that of the continuing ADVANCES IN CHEMISTRY SERIES except that, in order to save time, the papers are not typeset but are reproduced as they are submitted by the authors in camera-ready form. Papers are reviewed under the supervision of the Editors with the assistance of the Series Advisory Board and are selected to maintain the integrity of the symposia; however, verbatim reproductions of previously published papers are not accepted. Both reviews and reports of research are acceptable, because symposia may embrace both types of presentation.

Contents

Preface

THE DIVERSE CHEMICAL, BIOLOGICAL, AND INDUSTRIAL APPLICATIONS of the numerous synthetic carbon–fluorine compounds are almost legendary. In 1944, Marais identified fluoroacetate in the leaves of the South African shrub *Dichapetalum cymosum*; since then chemists and biologists continue to be intrigued by the natural occurrence, synthesis, and properties of the C–F bond.

A Ciba Foundation symposium was first published in 1972 to honor the contribution made by Sir Rudolph Peters to the biochemical aspects of the subject. This book was followed in 1976 by an ACS Symposium Series publication, *Biochemistry Involving Carbon–Fluorine Bonds*.

The natural occurrence of the C–F bond in carbohydrates is restricted to nucleocidin, an antibiotic in which the hydrogen at C-4 of this ribofuranoside is replaced by fluorine. In contrast, during the last 10 years, new synthetic methods for the introduction of both ^{19}F and ^{18}F into carbohydrates have led to an explosive growth in the number and variety of fluorinated sugars. Therefore, compounds that were relatively rare have become readily accessible for chemical and biochemical research.

The topics reported in this book reflect recent studies in the synthesis, reactivity, and some biochemical aspects of fluorinated carbohydrates. An appropriate combination of chemical and enzymatic methods now provides a versatile approach for the stereospecific introduction of fluorine into monosaccharides, disaccharides, oligosaccharides, and in the future, polysaccharides. A recurrent theme in biochemical studies is based on the rationale that ^{19}F and ^{18}F may replace the hydroxyl group of carbohydrates with minimal perturbance of molecular structure and conformation. The changes in biochemical reactivity, combined with the specific hydrogen-bonding capacity of the C–F bond, permit the use of deoxyfluorinated sugars as unique cellular and enzymatic probes. Studies illustrate carbohydrate metabolism, enzymology, antigen–antibody specificity, carbohydrate transport, and the design of new antiviral and antitumor agents. The inhibition and modification of viral-envelope glycoprotein synthesis by fluorinated sugars promises to be a new approach to the interference with virus—retrovirus—host cell membrane interactions.

The research reported in this volume raises more questions than it answers. For this reason, the future of fluorinated carbohydrates remains assured and many new avenues of research await further interdisciplinary investigation. I hope the chemical and biochemical scope of this book will continue to stimulate those already active in the field and attract new researchers into this exciting and fascinating area of carbohydrates.

Acknowledgments

I am deeply indebted to all contributors; without their patience and cooperation this book would not have been possible. I also wish to thank Robin Giroux and the staff of the ACS Books Department for guidance and assistance when it was most needed. Finally, my thanks to Donna Dee and Maeve Doyle for their expert secretarial and administrative assistance. Additional financial support for the organization of the symposium was kindly provided by E. I. du Pont de Nemours and Company.

N. F. TAYLOR
Department of Chemistry and Biochemistry
University of Windsor
Ontario N9B 3P4, Canada

January 1988

Chapter 1

Retrospect and Prospect

P. W. Kent

Nuffield Department of Clinical Biochemistry, Radcliffe Infirmary, Oxford University, Oxford, OX2 6HE, United Kingdom

In the past quarter of a century, interest has grown apace in these modified sugars, both in their chemistry as well as in their biological potentialities and a brief overview such as this can only touch on a few of the developments which have brought us to our present state of knowledge. For the most part, attention is devoted to monosaccharides containing a single F atom though undoubtedly others in which -CF$_3$ and -CF$_2$ have been introduced are both interesting and potentially important.

It was evident to early workers in the field that such F-sugars should be capable of existence if only on the grounds of the similarity of the F-atom to the OH group in size, electronegativity and ability to participate in H-bonded structures. Interest was further fuelled by the discovery of the high toxicity of monofluoro-acetate and by the bizarre fact that this compound occurred in Nature in many plants.

An extensive series of reviews of fluorinated biological analogues including F-carbohydrates was published in 1972 in the form of a CIBA Symposium volume (1) and an ACS Symposium in 1976 (2). A substantial, useful source book cataloguing properties of carbo-hydrate derivatives, including some fluorosugars has recently been published by Collins (3).

For brevity, F-sugar denotes a deoxyfluorocarbohydrate, eg. 6F-glucose denotes 6-deoxy-6-fluoro-D-glucose. This system is used throughout this chapter.

RETROSPECT

Like many other areas of organic chemistry, fluorocarbohydrates had small beginnings. The first tenuous tests seem to have been carried out by Moissan (4) himself, the discoverer of elemental fluorine. In his monumental monograph 'Fluor et ses Composés' published 1900, he wrote of the reaction between F$_2$ and glucose:

"Rien à froid: chauffé légèrment, il est attaqué par le fluor avec dépôt de charbon. Lorsque la temperature s'élève par suite de la réaction, la destruction devient

0097–6156/88/0374–0001$06.00/0

rapide et complète avec le fluoreuse de carbone et d'acide
fluorhydrique."

Sucrose and mannitol fared no better.

In the period to 1939, the limited means of synthesis led to a
slow accumulation of knowledge about fluoro-organic compounds and
their reactivity [a number of reviews of this earlier work were
published (5)]. Research in Poland, Belgium and Germany, in
particular, opened the way to further investigations. In the carbohydrate field, the most interesting findings were of the synthesis
and use of glycosyl fluorides with F at C1, which could be easily
obtained by exchange reactions with metallic fluorides or by the
action of liquid HF on fully acetylated monosaccharides. Results in
this field have been reviewed by Micheel and Klemer (6). These
derivatives provided a useful protecting group for C1, stable in
alkaline conditions but readily removable by dilute acids.

A curious finding made in connection with attempts to obtain
glucose from wood revealed that cellulose dissolved rapidly in
anhydrous HF to give glucosyl fluoride in high yield. If traces of
moisture were present, this product was not obtained and instead a
non-linear glucan, 'cellan', resulted (7). This was a random
structure, a highly branched polysaccharide in which several types
of interglycosidic linkages were present (8). Glucose itself could
be induced to polymerise in a variety of dehydrating acidic
conditions (eg. reference 9) to give a synthetic polysaccharide
with potential as a blood plasma extender.

During the period of World War II, much research was undertaken,
results of which were not published until 1947 and after, owing to
questions of national security. In particular studies were made of
fluorophosphidates [reviewed by Saunders (10)] and of derivatives of
fluoroacetic acid and its higher homologues [reviewed by Pattison
(11)].

The discovery in 1943 by Marais (12) that potassium fluoroacetate was the toxic material present in a number of South African
plants attracted notable attention, though the reasons for the
toxicity were not then known. Further exploration showed the
presence of the similarly toxic ω-fluorooleic acid in other plants.
At that time, the techniques for quantitative microanalysis of
organic fluorides were quite inadequate until an outstanding
complexometric method was devised in Belcher's laboratory (13). It
appeared from extensive surveys that fluorofatty acids in fact were
widespread in trace quantities in many species of green plants.

The biochemical mechanism of the toxicity of fluoroacetate in
mammals was first elucidated by the notable researches of the late
Sir Rudolph Peters, who showed that in liver and kidney, the compound
was metabolically transformed into an even more toxic fluorocitric
acid isomer, a powerful inhibitor of the tricarboxylic acid cycle.
These results together with those of others, Liébecq, Bergmann,
Buffa, Gál, to name but a few, established beyond doubt this new
biochemical twist in which a potential toxic agent could be transformed by an existing enzyme pathway into another of greater
toxicity creating a physiologically critical situation, a phenomenon
termed "Lethal Synthesis" by Peters.

With this in mind, it was even more challenging to pursue F-
carbohydrates to see whether these would be metabolised to yield

fluoroacetate as the end-product. Two principal approaches were
followed for their chemical synthesis; total syntheses and
fluorination of existing monosaccharide derivatives. The systematic
study of F-sugars was begun in Oxford in 1951 on these lines.

Total Syntheses

In this strategy, a simple starting compound, eg. ethyl fluoroacetate with the F-atom already positioned, equivalent in current
ideas to a synthon, was converted by Claisen condensation and
selective reduction into a number of simple F-analogues of
biochemical interest (Figure 1). By this route, 2F-glycerol and
2F-glyceric acid were obtained and like 1F-glycerol were found to be
metabolized to fluoroacetate and thus to be highly toxic. 2F-
Malate (2-hydroxy-3-fluoro(±)-butandioic acid) on the other hand
was relatively non-toxic despite its close structural relationship
to malic acid, a TCA cycle intermediate. In bacteria, it proved to
be a useful inducer of malate-utilising enzymes, however.

        2F-Erythritol (a competitive growth inhibitor of the *Brucella*
group) was a crystalline compound, isomorphous with erythritol
itself, whose structure had to be established by X-ray diffraction
analysis. 2F-Ribitol likewise was obtained by a similar synthetic
route.

        Total synthesis (14) however is a self-complicating route
generating multiple asymmetric centres which provides the investigator with a strong incentive to explore alternative strategies.

Modification of Monosaccharide Structures

Exchange Reactions.   Investigations had already been undertaken in
Helferich's laboratory which in 1941 (15) led to the synthesis of
6F-glucose by exchange of a sulphonyloxy ester by KF in methanol.
The sugar and its derivatives were obtained in good yield and
appeared to be stable. There was some fear at the time that loss
of HF by elimination might readily occur as a major side-reaction.

        In the 1950's further exploration of this route, modifying
solvent, blocking groups and conditions, led to 6F-galactose and a
number of monosaccharides F-substituted in the extra cyclic position.
Unlike the even-numbered ω-fluorofatty acids, none of these ω-
substituted sugars were metabolised to fluoroacetate and exhibited
little or no toxicity.

        Attempts to synthesise secondary 2-, 3- or 4-fluorosugars met
with little success. This was for a number of reasons such as
competing elimination reactions, the poor nucleophilicity of F^-,
the solvent dependence of the reaction, the availability of suitably
stable blocked sugars and the need to secure the appropriate axial
conformation of the departing ester group.

        These difficulties were progressively overcome by careful
systematic studies of the reaction conditions and by the introduction
of powerful new fluorinating agents. Amongst these tetrabutylammonium fluoride (Bu₄NF) was an outstanding discovery (16), as a
non-metallic ionic fluoride. By ingenious use of this reagent,
under rigorously anhydrous conditions, Foster and his group (17)
in 1967 achieved a synthesis of 3F-glucose (Figure 2). The method

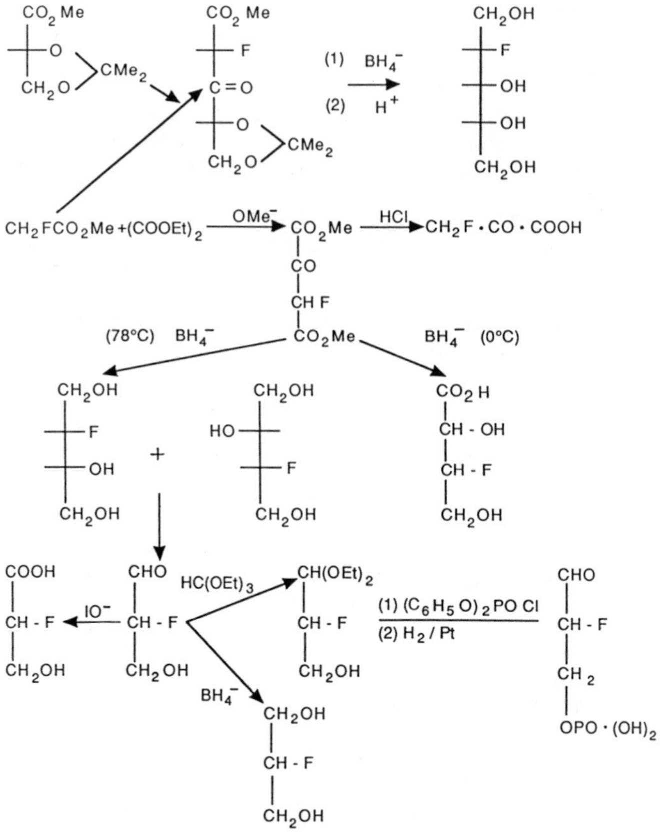

Figure 1. Total synthesis of three-, four- and five-carbon fluorosugars (all asymmetric products are racemic mixtures)

involved the oxidation of a glucose derivative with its equatorial
OH at C-3 to an oxo group which on BH_4^- reduction gave the axial OH
at C-3 favourable for F^- exchange of the CH_3SO_2 ester. This
important advance led to further secondary F-sugars, eg. 4F-glucose,
especially as O-methyl and O-benzyl groups came to be used for
protecting OH centres (18,19).

Further advances were made as a result of the signal discovery
by Middleton (20), of powerful new fluorinating agents, dialkylamino-
sulphur trifluoride (Et_2NSF_3 otherwise known as DAST) and
bis(dialkylamino) sulphur difluoride [$(Et_2N)_2SF_2$] as easily
handable reagents for replacing OH groups by F directly under mild
conditions. The conditions of the exchange were such that even O-
acetates provided adequate protection of the starting sugar. Sharma
and Korytnyk (21) thus obtained 6F-glucose by this method from
1,2,3,4-tetra-O-acetyl-glucose in good yield and without side
reactions.

This method proved to have wide application to secondary and
tertiary alcohol groups providing that the axial OH conformation is
attainable.

The approach has been further extended by researches in Szarek's
laboratory (22) which showed that tris(trimethylamino)sulphonium
difluorotrimethylsilicate (TSAF) (23) was another most effective
fluorinating agent for OH compounds.

The introduction of improved leaving groups such as $CF_3SO_3^-$
(triflate) led to the synthesis of 1F-fructose (24) and a range of
other secondary F-monosaccharides. These reactions proceed rapidly
and unambiguously under mild anhydrous conditions. This reaction
offers considerable promise for a fast means of introducing $^{18}F^-$
into biological analogues for positron emission transaxial tomography (PETT).

A number of reviews of exchange reactions and their products
have been published (25-27). The list of efficient fluorinating
agents continues to grow.

Epoxide Scission.   The success of parallel investigations in the
steroid field in obtaining fluoroderivatives by cleavage of epoxides
by HF and similar reagents even when secondary and tertiary centres
were involved gave considerable encouragement to applying the
method to sugar epoxides (28). The first practicable results were
obtained by Taylor and his coworkers (29) and by Bergmann's group
(30). These investigations led to 3F-xylose in good yield by
reaction of a 5-O-benzyl-2:3-anhydroriboside with HF or KHF_2 in
ethandiol. This was a significant breakthrough and this route
first led Pacák and coworkers (31) to the important probe compound,
2F-glucose.

Addition Reactions.   A further important synthetic route lay in
halogen and activated F donor addition to 1:2 glycoseens. Results
describing Br_2 and other halogen additions were already available
in the extensive and daunting paper by Fischer, Bergmann and Schotte
(32) published in 1920. Additions using interhalogens, 'BrF' and
'IF' (formed *in situ*) with triacetylglucal showed that the predominant products were the *gluco* and *manno* epimers of 2-deoxy-2-bromo
(or iodo)-glycosyl fluorides. The reaction was characteristically a

trans addition with F taking up the axial C-1 position and bromine
(or iodine) at C-2. The route was ineffective for fluorination at
other positions. The mechanism of this type of reaction in
accounting for the multiple isomeric products was substantially
elucidated by the elegant work of Lemieux, Frazer-Reid and
colleagues (33) and by pioneer development of ^{1}H and ^{19}F-NMR
techniques especially by L.D. Hall (34) and by R.A. Dwek (35).
    Signal success was obtained by the use of fluoro-oxytrifluoro-
methane (CF$_3$OF) introduced by Barton (36) in 1969. Carbohydrate
applications were undertaken in laboratories in London and Oxford.
It was shown (37) that CF$_3$OF reacted readily with triacetylglucal
at -78° giving chiefly the corresponding 2F-glucosyl α-glycoside
(34%) and its CF$_3$O α-glycoside (26%). In addition the corresponding
β-manno- compounds were present as minor products (Figure 3). This
was ascribed to the dismutation:

$$CF_3OF \rightleftharpoons CF_3O^- + F^+ \rightleftharpoons CF_2 = O + F_2$$

At the same time, comparable products resulted in the reactions with
triacetylgalactal, diacetylxylal and diacetylarabinal (38-40).
Conformational effects arising from the configuration of the
substituent at C-4 played a significant role in controlling the
stereochemistry of addition products (41) such as those arising
from diacetylrhamnal (42), diacetylfucal (43) and heptacetyl-lactal
(44).
    Progress in the field was greatly aided by results from Wolf's
laboratory (45,46) in 1977 on the direct fluorination of triacetylglucal with F$_2$. Conditions were found in which a rapid and
controlled reaction took place giving the 2F-glucosyl α-fluoride
(40% yield) and the 2F-mannosyl β-fluoride (26%) derivatives.
These results proved to be of utmost value for the synthesis of the
^{18}F-labelled compounds for positron emission tomography. The speed
with which the addition and subsequent separations could be achieved
experimentally enabled the 2-^{18}F-glucose to be obtained with a radio-
active purity of over 98% and with high specific activity, eg.
8750 mCi/mmol. The labelled sugar has come into extensive
prominence for the mapping in vivo of regions of elevated glucose
requirements as indicative of tissue abnormalities. The biochemical
comparability of 2F-glucose, its apparent non-toxicity and the
short half-life of the isotope (^{18}F, t$_{\frac{1}{2}}$ 110 mins) offers distinctive
suitability for non-invasive diagnostic use by PETT.

Some Biological Effects

Though in animals F-monosaccharides are rarely if ever metabolised
to F-acetate, nevertheless they enter into a number of biochemical
pathways including oxidation, primary phosphorylation by kinases and
conversion into nucleotide F-sugar phosphates, thence to make their
appearance in a number of glycoproteins and glycolipids.
    Schmidt, Schwarz and colleagues (47,48) further showed that 2F-
mannose and 2F-glucose inhibited the biosyntheses of infective
Semliki virus and fowl plague virus (influenza virus A) in chick
embryo cells and that of pseudorabies virus in rabbit kidney cells.
This was attributed to failure to complete the viral envelope (49)

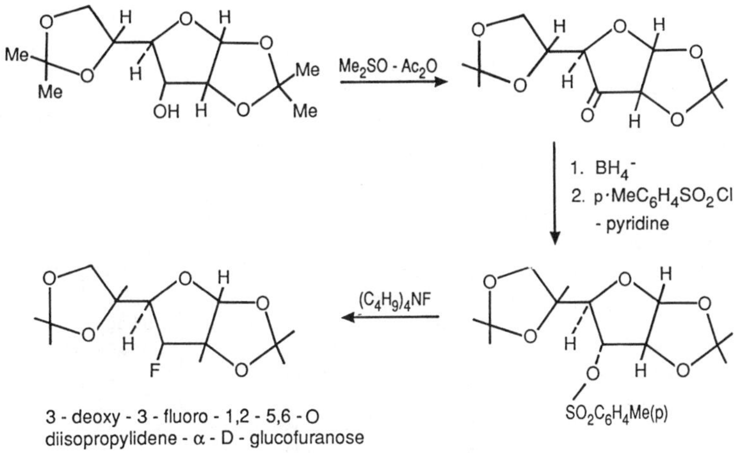

3 - deoxy - 3 - fluoro - 1,2 - 5,6 - O
diisopropylidene - α - D - glucofuranose

Figure 2. Synthesis of 3-deoxy-3-fluoro-D-glucose

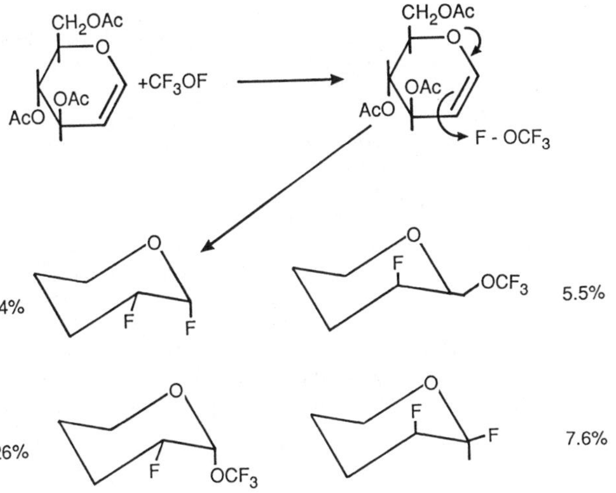

Figure 3. Addition of CF_3OF to 3,4,6-tri-*O*-acetyl-D-glucal

in a manner analogous to 2-deoxyglucose (2DG) which underwent conversion via the GDP intermediate to give a chain-terminating lipid 2DG(GlcNAc)$_2$PP Dolichol. The inhibition was relieved by addition of mannose. The blocked lipid was incapable of mannosylation required for formation of N-linked oligosaccharide components in appropriate glycoproteins.

These 2F-sugars caused extensive oligosaccharide chain-shortening in glycolipids of influenza A infected chick cells and in yeast (50). The alteration in membrane molecular architecture consequent on these modifications points to substantial prospects for reducing viral infectivity, as Blough and Giuntoli (51) found in the treatment of human genital herpes with 2DG. The field was reviewed in 1982 by Schwarz and Datema (52).

Amongst the glycosaminoglycans, N-fluoro[³H]acetyl-D-glucosamine and N-fluoroacetyl-D-[1-¹⁴C]glucosamine was found (53) to be incorporated into hyaluronate by mammalian cells, via the UDP-intermediates (54). The resulting hyaluronate containing N-fluoro-acetylglucosaminyl residues, ³H-labelled in the N-substituent and 1-¹⁴C-ring labelled, appeared to be more resistant to hyaluronidase degradation than the fluorine-free counterpart from the same tissue, suggesting that carbohydrate complexes, biosynthetically modified in this fashion, may have extended half-lives *in vivo*.

2F-Glucose and other F-monosaccharides can promote reduction in cell growth of a number of tumour cell lines in culture (55,56) but appear to have little effect on tumours *in vivo*. In murine lymphoma cells, 2F-glucose was an effective growth inhibitor, while N-trifluoroacetyl-D-glucosamine diminished the incorporation of glucosamine into cell components. The underlying mechanisms to account for growth inhibition are considered to be due in part to metabolic imbalance between intracellular pools of critical biochemical intermediates, as well as by the cell surface modifications. Disturbance of glycoprotein structure has also been achieved by depletion of glycosylation through metabolic incorporation of threo β-fluoroasparagine into the polypeptide sequence thus denying N-glycosylation [reviewed by Elbein (57)].

A further important mechanism affecting mammalian cell metabolism was found by Barnett (58) in sugar transport phenomena. In the mammalian intestinal mucosa and in the red cell, 3F-glucose, for example, was a specific competitive inhibitor of the transport of the parent sugar. Cells grown in the presence of sub-limiting concentrations of the 3F-sugar experienced glucose deprivation and carbohydrate starvation with consequent restriction in cell growth. Interestingly, α-D-glucopyranosyl fluoride proved to be a substrate for intestinal α-glucosidase, a substrate with the smallest aglycone possible.

In non-mammalian systems, F-sugars have other biochemical properties. For example, 3F-glucose is oxidized in *Pseudomonas putida* to F-aldonic acids (59), whereas 4F-glucose is metabolized only after cleavage of the C-F bond by an outer membrane protein (60). The end product of this reaction has been identified as 4,5-dihydroxypentanoic acid (61). In *Locusta migratoria*, Taylor has shown a further unusual metabolic degradation of 3F-glucose with liberation of F⁻. The incorporation of 3F-glucose into trehalose and into modified glycogen was also shown to occur (62).

PROSPECT

The ease with which F-monosaccharides can now be synthesized by relatively straightforward chemical or chemoenzymatic (63) methods makes this class of sugar attractive in many areas of research.

To the synthetic organic chemist, these compounds offer a range of starting materials, with one or more fluorine atoms stereochemically specified, suitable for the chiron methods of assembly (64) of more complex molecules. Design of retro-synthetic routes could enable precise fluoro-analogues of hormones, surface-active lipids and vitamins for example to be synthesized with a view to seeking agents of enhanced biological activity and of longer retention time *in vivo*. It will be recalled that 9-α-fluorocortisol is a well known instance amongst the steroid hormones of such enhancement.

There is also substantial promise in semi-synthetic approaches where, with ever-improving methods for fluorinating specific molecular sites in existing natural products, new and potentially important molecular modifications can be envisaged. The possibilities which may be opened by introducing even a single F-atom at a crucial position in, say, the penicillins, tetracyclins or cephalosporins are immense especially as the questions of microbial resistance become the more pressing. One notes the existence of at least one naturally occurring antibiotic, nucleocidin (65) containing an F-atom attached to C4 of a ribofuranosyl residue. Beginnings have been made using F-sugar derivatives as anti-viral agents and the possibilities of influencing *in vivo* their growth and infectivity specifically and with minimal disturbance to the host hold out great promise (66).

A further aspect of these possibilities is in relation to the powerful new non-invasive imaging techniques which NMR and PETT (67) offer and no doubt even more powerful techniques will follow in the future. The NMR distinctive chemical shifts arising from ^{19}F suggest that methods are realisable for locating F-containing pharmacological agents *in vivo* and possibly for their pharmacodynamic investigation. *In vivo* probes as well as those *in vitro* can be envisaged as leading to new understanding of membrane binding and retention of selectively transported molecules.

The central enigma of the biochemical means by which the C-F bond is synthesized still remains unsolved even in outline. Though this is assumed to be a phenomenon restricted to plants, this may not be wholly the case. Not only is the origin of F-acetate ripe for reinvestigation but also that of volatile plant products such as FCH_2COCH_3 and $FCH_2CH_2OCH_2CH_3$. Whatever the pathway of F-acetate formation, it can be presumed to be an unusual one and may be of substantial interest to the inorganic chemist. It is interesting to speculate whether a fluoro-silicon intermediate is involved which participates in an exchange with an activated phosphate ester. The question is only marginally relevant to F-sugars at the present time however.

To the biochemist and physiologist, fluoro-containing biological analogues are of great potential interest. The development of routes for the biological incorporation of F-sugars into strategic biopolymers is particularly so. For example, it is of

interest to explore in much greater detail the possible role of
4F-glucose in glycogen synthesis and glycogenolysis, where even
partial incorporation of the F-sugar can be envisaged as a chain-
terminating step in outer-branch chains of the molecule. In
glycogen storage diseases, where over-production and deposition of
the polysaccharide occurs, the approach could be a valuable one.
And a range of other storage diseases await investigation.

The more complex chemical structures and biological recognition
sites amongst the glycoproteins in some cases mediated through cell
surface oligosaccharides, presents legion possibilities for similar
metabolic intervention by introduction of F-sugars or deoxysugars.
Mild and selective fluorination methods may come here to have
importance in semi-synthetic modifications of pre-existing proteins,
glycoproteins and polypeptides. Again the possibility of increasing
in vivo the retention time in circulation, points to ways of
reducing the dose levels of administered therapeutic agents and
perhaps of targeting them more accurately to designated tissues.

The progress in the field in the last quarter of a century
has been impressive but many more exciting developments yet await us.

Acknowledgments

I thank Dr. G.E. Newman and Mrs. Jean Smith for their help in
preparing this chapter.

Literature Cited

1. CIBA Symposium, Carbon-Fluorine Compounds: Chemistry,
    Biochemistry and Biological Activities; Associated Scientific
    Publishers: Amsterdam, 1972.
2. Biochemistry Involving Carbon Fluorine Bonds: Filler, R. (ed.);
    ACS Symposium Series 28, American Chemical Society, Washington,
    D.C., 1976, 1-214.
3. Collins, P.M. Carbohydrates; Chapman Hall: London, U.K., 1987.
4. Moissan, H. Le Fluor et ses Composés; G. Steinheil: Paris, 1900;
    p.244.
5. (i) Lovelace, A.M.; Rausch, D.A.; Postelnek, W. Aliphatic
        Fluorine Compounds; Reinhold Publishing Corp.: New York,
        1958.
   (ii) Hudlický, M. Chemistry of Organic Fluorine Compounds;
        Pergamon Press: Oxford, U.K., 1961.
   (iii)New Methods of Preparative Organic Chemistry; Interscience
        Publications Inc.: New York, 1948 (English translation of
        German researches published in 1944) Bockemüller, W.,
        pp.229-45 and Weichert, K., pp.315-62.
6. Micheel, F.; Klemer, A. Adv. Carbohydr. Chem. 1961, 16, 85-103.
7. Fredenhagen, K.; Cadenbach, G. Angew. Chem. 1933, 46, 113-117.
8. Helferich, B.; Peters, O. Annalen 1932, 494, 101-106, and
    references therein.
9. Pacsu, E.; Mora, P.T. J. Am. Chem. Soc. 1950, 72, 1045.
10. Saunders, B.C. Some Aspects of the Chemistry and Toxic Action
    of Organic Compounds containing Phosphorus and Fluorine;
    Cambridge University Press: Cambridge, U.K., 1957.
11. Pattison, F.L.M. Toxic Aliphatic Fluorine Compounds; Elsevier
    Publishing Co.: Amsterdam, 1959.

12. Marais, J.S.C. Onderstepoort J. Vet. Sci. Anim. Ind. 1943, 18, 203-206.
13. Belcher, R.; Leonard, M.A.; West, T.S. J. Chem. Soc., 1959, 3577-79.
14. Zamojski, A.; Banaszek, A.; Grynkiewicz, G. Adv. Carbohydr. Chem. Biochem. 1982, 40, 1-20.
15. Helferich, B.; Gnüchtel, A. Chem. Ber. 1941, 74, 1035-39.
16. Henbest, H.B.; Jackson, W.R. J. Chem. Soc. 1962, 954-59.
17. Foster, A.B.; Hems, R.; Webber, J.M. Carbohydr. Res. 1967, 5, 292-301.
18. Foster, A.B.; Hems, R.; Westwood, J.M. Carbohydr. Res. 1970, 15, 41-49.
19. Lopes, D.P.; Taylor, N.F. Carbohydr. Res. 1979, 73, 125-134.
20. Middleton, W.J. J. Org. Chem. 1975, 40, 547-78.
21. Sharma, M.; Korytnyk, W. Tetrahedron Letters 1977, 6, 573-76.
22. Szarek, W.A.; Hay, G.W.; Doboszewski, B. Chem. Comm. 1985, 663-64.
23. Middleton, W.J. U.S. Patent 3 940 402, 1976.
24. Card, P.J.; Hitz, W.D. J. Am. Chem. Soc. 1984, 106, 5348-50.
25. Barnett, J.E.G. Adv. Carbohydr. Chem. Biochem. 1967, 22, 177-227.
26. Penglis, A.A.E. Adv. Carbohydr. Chem. Biochem. 1981, 38, 195-285.
27. Kent, P.W. in CIBA Symposium, Carbon-Fluorine Compounds: Chemistry, Biochemistry and Biological Activities; Associated Scientific Publishers: Amsterdam, 1972, pp.168-208.
28. Taylor, N.F.; Kent, P.W. Adv. Fluorine Chem. 1963, 4, 113-141.
29. Taylor, N.F.; Childs, R.F.; Brunt, R.V. Chem. & Ind. 1964, 928-929.
30. Cohen, S.; Levy, D.; Bergmann, E.D. Chem. & Ind. 1964, 1802-3.
31. Pacák, J.; Tocík, Z.; Cerný, M. Chem. Comm. 1969, 77.
32. Fischer, E.; Bergmann, M.; Schotte, H. Chem. Ber. 1920, 53B, 509-47.
33. Lemieux, R.U.; Frazer-Reid, B. Can. J. Chem. 1965, 43, 1460-75.
34. Hall, L.D.; Manville, J.F.; Bhacca, N.S. Can. J. Chem. 1969, 47, 1-18.
35. Dwek, R.A. in CIBA Symposium, Carbon-Fluorine Compounds: Chemistry, Biochemistry and Biological Activities; Associated Scientific Publishers: Amsterdam, 1972, pp.239-71.
36. Barton, D.R.H.; Danko, L.J.; Ganguly, A.K.; Hesse, R.H.; Tarzia, G.; Pecket, M.M. Chem. Comm. 1969, 227.
37. Adamson, J.; Foster, A.B.; Hall, L.D.; Hesse, R.H. Chem. Comm. 1969, 309-310.
38. Dwek, R.A.; Kent, P.W.; Kirby, P.T.; Harrison, A.S. Tetrahedron Letters 1970, 2987-90.
39. Butchard, G.C.; Kent, P.W. Tetrahedron 1971, 27, 3457-63.
40. Adamson, I.; Marcus, D.M. Carbohydr. Res. 1970, 13, 314-16.
41. Evelyn, L.; Hall, L.D. Carbohydr. Res. 1976, 47, 285-97.
42. Butchard, G.C.; Kent, P.W. Tetrahedron 1975, 35, 2439-43.
43. Butchard, G.C.; Kent, P.W. Tetrahedron 1975, 35, 2551-54.
44. Kent, P.W.; Dimitrijevich, S.D. J. Fluorine Chem. 1977, 10, 455-78.
45. Ido, T.; Wan, C-N.; Fowler, J.S.; Wolf, A.P. J. Org. Chem. 1977, 42, 2431-32.

46. Ido, T.; Wan, C-N.; Casella, V.; Fowler, J.S.; Wolf, A.P.; Reivich, M.; Kuhl, D.E. J. Labelled Compounds & Radiopharmaceuticals 1978, 19, 173-183.
47. Schmidt, M.G.; Schwarz, R.T.; Ludwig, H. J. Virol. 1976, 18, 819-23.
48. Schmidt, M.G.; Biely, P.; Kratz, Z.; Schwarz, R.T. Eur. J. Biochem. 1978, 87, 55-68.
49. Schwarz, R.T.; Schmidt, M.G.; Datema, R. Biochem. Soc. Trans. 1979, 7, 322-26.
50. Datema, R.; Schwarz, R.T. Biochem. J. 1979, 184, 113-123.
51. Blough, H.A.; Giuntoli, R.L. J. Am. Med. Soc. Ass. 1979, 241, 2798-2801.
52. Schwarz, R.T.; Datema, R. Adv. Carbohydr. Chem. Biochem. 1982, 40, 287-379.
53. Winterbourne, D.J.; Barnby, R.; Mian, N.; Kent, P.W. Biochem. J. 1979, 182, 707-16.
54. Schulz, A.M.; Mora, P.T. Carbohydr. Res. 1975, 40, 119-127.
55. Bernacki, R.J.; Sharma, M.; Porter, N.K.; Rustum, Y.; Paul, B.; Korytnyk, W. J. Supermol. Structure 1977, 7, 235-50.
56. Paul, B.; Korytnyk, W. in Cell Surface Carbohydrate Chemistry; Academic Press: New York, 1978; pp.311-35.
57. Elbein, A.D. Ann. Rev. Biochem. 1987, 56, 497-534.
58. Barnett, J.E.G. in CIBA Symposium, Carbon-Fluorine Compounds: Chemistry, Biochemistry and Biological Activities; Associated Scientific Publishers: Amsterdam, 1972, pp.95-109.
59. Taylor, N.F.; Hill, L.; Eisenthal, R. Can. J. Biochem. 1975, 53, 57-64.
60. D'Amore, T.; Taylor, N.F. FEBS Lett. 1982, 143, 247-51.
61. Sbrissa, D.; McIntosh, J.M.; Taylor, N.F. Proc. Can Fed. Biol. Soc. Abstr. 1987, 30, 141.
62. Agbanyo, M.; Taylor, N.F. Bioscience Reports 1986, 6, 309-16.
63. Drueckhammer, D.G.; Wong, C-H. J. Org. Chem. 1985, 50, 5912-13.
64. Henessian, S. Total Synthesis of Natural Products: The 'Chiron' Approach; Pergamon Press: Oxford, U.K., 1983.
65. Morton, G.O.; Lancaster, J.E.; Van Lear, G.E.; Fulmor, W.; Meyer, W.E. J. Am. Chem. Soc. 1969, 91, 1535-37.
66. Leyland-Jones, B.; Donnelly, H.; Groshen, S.; Myskowski, P.; Fox, J.J. J. Infectious Dis. 1987, 154, 430-36.
67. Dagani, R. Chem. & Eng. News 1981, 9 Nov., 30-37.

RECEIVED January 8, 1988

Chapter 2

Preparation and Reactions of Glycosyl Fluorides

Jared L. Randall[1] and K. C. Nicolaou

Department of Chemistry, University of Pennsylvania, Philadelphia, PA 19104

In recent years, fluorinated carbohydrates have been studied intensively, both as biochemical probes and as glycosylating agents. In this paper, the preparation and reactions of glycosyl fluorides will be reviewed with emphasis on the use of glycosyl fluorides prepared from thioglycosides. Applications of this technology to the synthesis of carbohydrate - containing natural products will be presented. Additionally, the novel 1,2-migration reaction induced by diethylaminosulfur trifluoride (DAST) will be discussed.

Although fluorinated carbohydrates have been a subject of interest for decades (1), the recent realization ·that glycosyl fluorides can be synthetically useful has sparked renewed investigation in this area. The modern advances in the preparation and reactions of glycosyl fluorides have been surveyed recently in an extensive review (2); therefore, this lecture will focus on the use of glycosyl fluorides in natural product synthesis and the studies carried out in our laboratories.

Preparation of Glycosyl Fluorides

The review by Card (2) concisely presents the variety of reported methods for the preparation of glycosyl fluorides from a number of precursors. Although they have been prepared from glycosyl chlorides, acetates, and pivaloates and glycoses, we have found thioglycosides to be more versatile precursors to glycosyl fluorides. The employment of thioglycosides allows the selective activation of the anomeric center early in the synthetic scheme, obviating the selective deprotection or activation of the anomeric center directly before fluorination.
    The Nicolaou group's interest in the development of mild methods for the formation of O-glycosidic linkages to complex natural

[1]Current address: The Procter and Gamble Company, Miami Valley Laboratories, P.O. Box 398707, Cinncinnati, OH 45239–8707

0097–6156/88/0374–0013$06.00/0
o 1988 American Chemical Society

products led to investigations of glycosyl fluorides as glycosyl donors. The key discovery that led to these applications was the realization that phenyl thioglycosides can be efficiently converted to glycosyl fluorides (Figure 1) (3). Treatment of phenyl thioglycosides (1) with diethylaminosulfur trifluoride (DAST) or hydrogen fluoride-pyridine complex (HF-pyr), and N-bromosuccinimide (NBS) in dichloromethane at -15-0°C provides glycosyl fluorides (3) in good to excellent yields. Additionally, it was found that many protecting groups, which cannot withstand the more drastic conditions commonly used for glycosyl donor formation, tolerate these conditions; indeed, even silyl ethers are stable to the reaction conditions when DAST is utilized as the fluorinating agent.

It is reasonable to assume that this fluorination reaction proceeds via an intermediate bromosulfonium ion (2, Figure 1) which is attacked by a fluoride ion. The fluoride ion donor ability of HF-pyridine complex is well known; however, in this case the mechanism by which DAST is able to donate the fluoride ion is not as straightforward. We propose two possible mechanisms by which this reaction may proceed (Figure 2). Mechanism A involves the succinimide ion which is formed as a byproduct in the bromination reaction. The succinimide ion may attack the sulfur atom in the DAST reagent and displace a fluoride ion which, in turn, opens the bromo-sulphonium ion (4). An alternative mechanism (B) involves the lone pair of electrons in the DAST reagent which displaces the fluoride ion which then attacks the bromosulphonium species (5). The second mechanism seems more plausible in view of the fact that this reaction, in most cases, proceeds to completion very quickly.

Reactions of Glycosyl Fluorides

The use of glycosyl fluorides as glycosyl donors is advantageous for the synthetic chemist because, they are readily prepared, stable to column chromatography, and tolerant of storage for extended periods of time. Until recently, glycosyl fluorides were considered to be too stable for use as glycosyl donors (1). However, the advent of the Mukaiyama conditions for the formation of the O-glycosidic linkage generated intensive study of the reactions of glycosyl fluorides (2,4). After surveying many activating agents, Mukaiyama and coworkers found that utilizing a combination of silver perchlorate and stannous chloride as promoters converted β-glycosyl fluorides to O-glycosides in high yields and with good α-glycoside selectivities.

We have found the Mukaiyama reaction to be extremely useful and have extended the application of this method to the selective synthesis of β-glycosides as well as α-glycosides. By taking advantage of solvent effects and protecting groups at the 2-position, remarkable stereoselectivity in the formation of O-glycosidic linkages has been obtained (5). Once the optimum conditions were ascertained, the anomeric configuration of the glycosyl fluoride was not found to have any significant effect on the stereoselectivity of the glycosidation reaction (3). This phenomenon has also been reported by Ogawa et al. (6,7). We concur with these investigators' proposition that the high stereoselectivity of these reactions is due to the formation of intimate ion pairs, as previously proposed by Lemieux (8) and Paulsen (9) for other glycosyl donors.

When used in conjunction with the mild preparation of glycosyl fluorides from thioglycosides, the Mukaiyama conditions provide the key to a mild, selective method for the synthesis of the O-glycosidic linkage. We have found this method to be practicable for the formation of glycoside bonds to sensitive, complex aglycones and for the repetitive, block-type syntheses of oligosaccharides. The use of thioglycosides as precursors to glycosyl fluorides is keenly suited for these applications because the thioglycoside functionality can: 1) be used to mask the anomeric center early in the synthetic scheme; 2) exist in the glycosyl acceptor without interfering with the glycosidation reaction; and 3) when desired, be converted to the glycosyl fluoride under mild conditions.

Formation of O-Glycosidic Linkages to Sensitive Aglycones. The first application of this technology to natural products synthesis was the partial synthesis of avermectin B$_{1a}$ (3).The oleandrose derivative (6, Figure 3) was prepared from L-rhamnose and converted to glycosyl fluoride (7) in 80% yield by reaction with NBS and DAST. Removal of the silyl ether protecting group of the thioglycoside (6) afforded the hydroxyl component (8). Coupling of these two components, utilizing the Mukaiyama conditions, selectively provided the α-linked disaccharide (9). The disaccharide was then converted to glycosyl fluoride (10) (α:β ratio = 5:1) in 85% yield by treatment with NBS and DAST. Coupling of the disaccharide glycosyl donor to the avermectin aglycone derivative proceeded with complete α-anomeric selectivity in 62% yield. Desilylation of the resultant product provided avermectin B$_{1a}$. This synthesis demonstrates the synthetic utility of the method for the formation of O-glycosidic linkages to complex, sensitive aglycones.

Our method was also employed in the total synthesis of efrotomycin (10). The desired carbohydrate units (11 and 12, Figure 4) were efficiently prepared from D-allose and L-rhamnose, respectively. Conversion of the rhamnose-derived thioglycoside (12) to the corresponding glycosyl fluoride (13) was accomplished in 88% yield with the NBS/DAST conditions. By employing the Mukaiyama conditions, this glycosyl fluoride was efficiently coupled with glycosyl acceptor (11) in 75% yield to provide disaccharide (14) with total α-anomeric selectivity. But, when the thioglycoside obtained (14) was converted to the glycosyl fluoride (15) with the NBS/DAST conditions and coupled with goldinolactone (18), the undesired α-anomeric product was obtained. Nevertheless, protecting group interchange of the silyl protecting groups to neighboring-group-active acetyl groups provided disaccharide (16). After conversion of this disaccharide to glycosyl fluoride (17), coupling to goldinolactone allowed the preparation of the desired β-glycoside (19), exclusively, in 86% yield. This intermediate was then further elaborated to provide the first total synthesis of efrotomycin.

Synthesis of Oligosaccharides. To demonstrate the effectiveness of this technology for the repetitive and block-type synthesis of oligosaccharides, we targeted the linear hexasaccharide (28, Figure 5) consisting of six glucose units linked in an α(1→6) fashion (3). From the readily prepared phenyl thioglycoside (20), both the glycosyl fluoride (22, NBS/DAST, 90%, α:β ratio = 1:1) and the glyco-

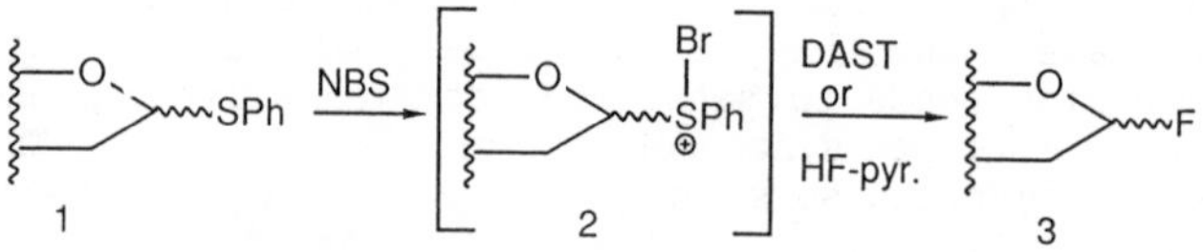

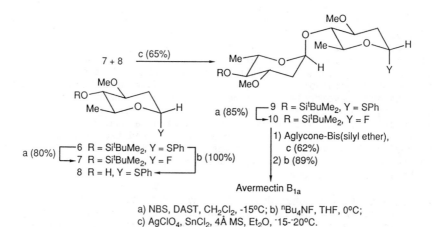

Figure 1. Formation of Glycosyl Fluorides from Thioglycosides.

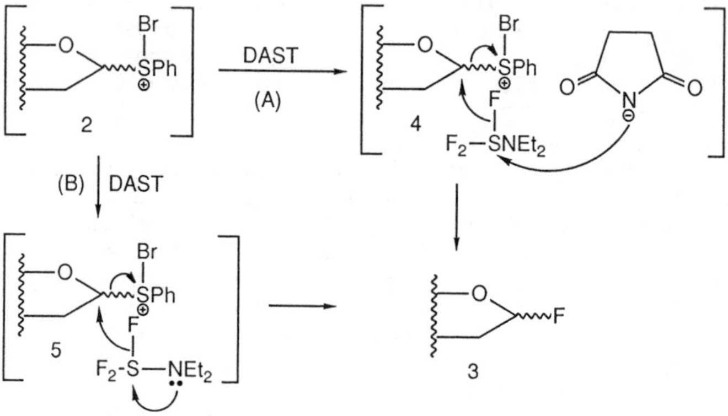

Figure 2. The Mechanism of the DAST Reaction.

a) NBS, DAST, CH₂Cl₂, -15°C; b) ⁿBu₄NF, THF, 0°C;
c) AgClO₄, SnCl₂, 4Å MS, Et₂O, ⁻15-⁻20°C.

Figure 3. Partial Synthesis of Avermectin B₁ₐ. (Adapted from Ref. 3.)

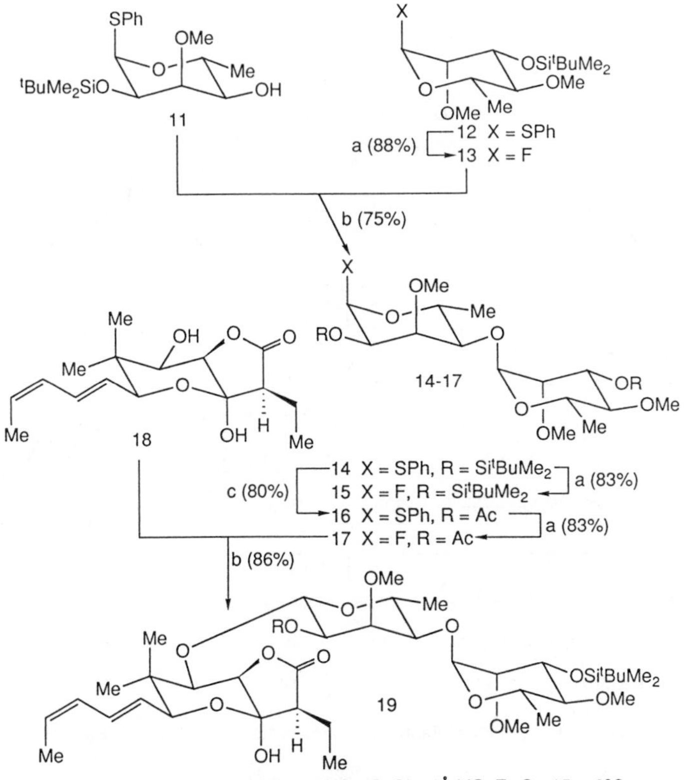

a) NBS, DAST, CH$_2$Cl$_2$, -15°C; b) AgClO$_4$, SnCl$_2$, 4Å MS, Et$_2$O, -15— 0°C;
c) i) ^{n}Bu$_4$NF, THF, 0-25°C, ii) Ac$_2$O, DMAP, CH$_2$Cl$_2$, 25°C.

Figure 4.   Attachment of the Carbohydrate Portion of
Efrotomycin.(Adapted from Ref. 10.)

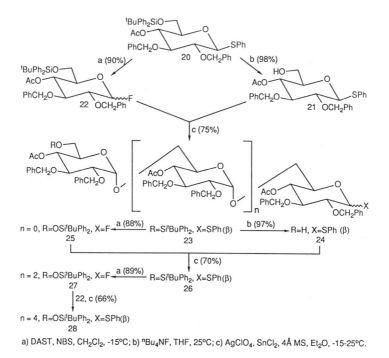

a) DAST, NBS, CH₂Cl₂, -15°C; b) ⁿBu₄NF, THF, 25°C; c) AgClO₄, SnCl₂, 4Å MS, Et₂O, -15-25°C.

Figure 5.   Synthesis of a Hexasaccharide.(Adapted from Ref. 3.)

syl acceptor (21, nBu₄NF, 90%) were obtained. Reaction of the two components under the Mukaiyama conditions provided predominantly the α-linked disaccharide (23, 75%, α:β ratio = 95:5). The small amount of the β-linked product was removed by flash column chromatography. Repetition of the fluorination and deprotection operations utilizing this disaccharide provided glycosyl fluoride (25, α:β ratio = 1:1) and glycosyl acceptor (24), respectively. Again, coupling of the two components, utilizing the Mukaiyama conditions, provided tetrasaccharide (26) (α:β ratio = 95:5), and after conversion to the glycosyl fluoride and coupling to the disaccharide glycosyl acceptor (24), the hexasaccharide (28, α:β ratio = 95:5) was obtained.

The synthesis of the hexasaccharide demonstrates that our new technology provides a convenient, efficient method for the synthesis of oligosaccharides. The most noteworthy feature of our procedure that makes it particularly suited for these operations is the ability to selectively and efficiently activate the anomeric position under mild conditions; additionally, by coupling the glycosyl fluoride with a thioglycoside glycosyl acceptor, the stage is set for the process to be effectively repeated.

Synthesis of the Rhynchosporosides. Having established the synthetic viability of this method for the synthesis of oligosaccharides, we sought to apply the technology to natural products synthesis. We targeted a series of oligosaccharide phytotoxins, the rhynchosporosides, and devised a convergent, general synthetic scheme that would utilize common intermediates for the preparation of each of the oligomers (5). For example, in the synthesis of the pentasaccharide oligomer bearing the aglycone with the R-configuration, which we have termed the [5R]-rhynchosporoside, our technology proved to be highly effective (Figure 6).

The required tetrasaccharide (33) was prepared from cellobiosyl fluoride (29, α:β ratio = 1:3) by successive addition of two glucose units. By coupling the cellobiose derivative with the monosaccharide building block (30, AgClO₄, SnCl₂, 75%), conversion of the resultant product to the glycosyl fluoride (NBS, DAST, 85%, α:β ratio = 1:1), and repetition of the two step process, the tetrasaccharide building block was obtained. The neighboring-group-active acetyl group allowed the selective formation of the β(1→4) linkage. In each of the coupling reactions, only the desired β-anomer was isolated; any small amounts of α-linked products were beyond the limits of detection.

The tetrasaccharide glycosyl donor was coupled to the protected glucoside unit with the protected glycerol unit already in place. This terminal unit was prepared from glucosyl fluoride (35, α:β ratio = 2:1) which was suitibly protected with the neighboring-group-inactive benzyl group. Coupling of this glycosyl fluoride with the protected glycerol unit (36) using the Mukaiyama conditions, followed by deacetylation, provided the α-linked product exclusively in 75% overall yield. Coupling of the oligosaccharide chain with the terminal monosaccharide moiety provided the fully protected [5R]-rhynchosporoside in 72% yield. Deprotection of the pentasaccharide by desilylation, deacetylation and debenzylation provided the natural product in excellent overall yield. This synthesis demonstrates the synthetic utility of our method for the repetitive, block-type syn-

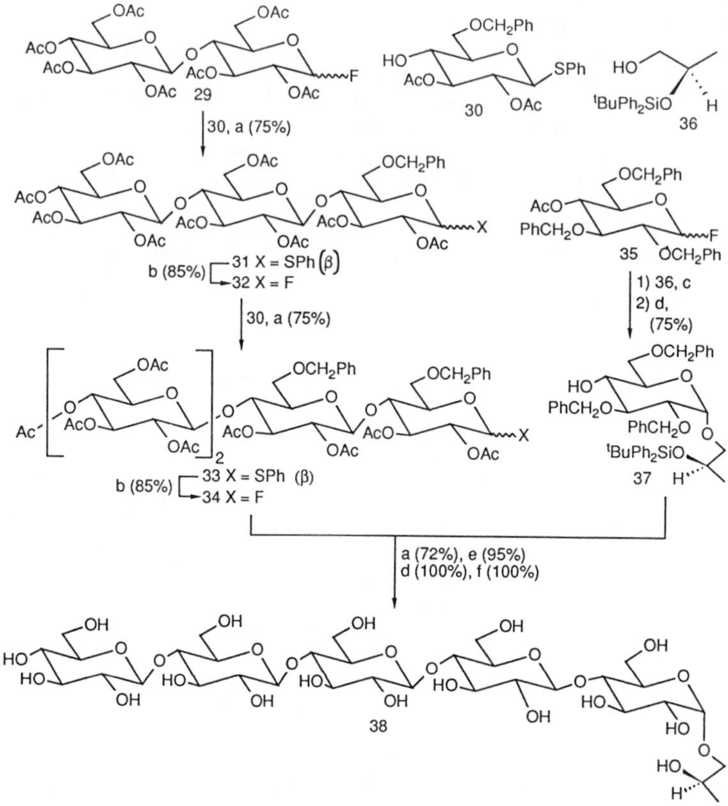

a) AgClO₄, SnCl₂, 4Å MS, CH₂Cl₂, ⁻15-⁻20°C; b) NBS, DAST, CH₂Cl₂, 0°C; c) AgClO₄, SnCl₂, 4Å MS, Et₂O, ⁻15-⁻20°C; d) NaOMe, MeOH, 25°C; e) HF-pyr, THF, 0°C; f) H₂, Pd(OH)₂/C, MeOH, H₂O, 25°C.

Figure 6.   Synthesis of the [5R]-Rhynchosporoside. (Adapted from Ref. 5.)

theses that are often required in the preparation of oligosaccharide natural products.

Other Studies of Glycosyl Fluorides in Natural Product Synthesis. Besides the studies carried out in our laboratories, there are few examples of the utilization of glycosyl fluorides as glycosyl donors in the synthesis of natural products. However, Ogawa et al. have recently reported the use of glycosyl fluorides in the synthesis of a heptasaccharide hapten (6), the Le^b antigen (11), and globotriaosyl ceramides (12), but other glycosyl donors were also utilized in these syntheses.

One of this group's most recent publications describes a thorough study of the formation of α(1→4) oligogalactosides from glycosyl fluorides (7). For example, as shown in Figure 7, they investigated the reaction of galactobiosyl fluoride (39) with glycosyl acceptor (40) under the Mukaiyama conditions and found that the α-glycoside (41) as obtained exclusively in 89% yield. They reasoned that, due to the exo-anomeric effect (13), the molecule was in the conformation essentially depicted in Figure 7; therefore, attack of the hydroxyl group of the glycosyl donor on the intimate ion pair, from the convex face of the molecule, was predisposed to give the α-glycoside. More in-depth studies on the glycosylation reactions of glycosyl fluorides, such as this one, are needed to fully understand the reactivity of these glycosyl donors.

Other Reactions of Glycosyl Fluorides

We (14) and others (15) have found that C-, O-, S- and N-glycosides can be readily prepared from glycosyl fluorides. For example, in many cases we found boron trifluoride-etherate to be an effective promoter for these applications, as shown in Figure 8 (14). For the preparation of C- and N-glycosides, trimethylsilyl derivatives were shown to be effective nucleophiles (entries 1 and 2). Glycosyl phosphate esters may be formed in moderate yields by activation of the glycosyl acceptors as stannyl ethers (entry 3). In other investigations with boron trifluoride-etherate, it was discovered that thiols and carboxylic acids could be efficiently coupled without further activation. In some cases, activation of glycosyl acceptors with trimethylaluminum allowed the formation of glycoside derivatives without the addition of other promoters. This reaction could be utilized for the preparation of C-glycosides and glycosyl amines. These investigations demonstrate the versatility of glycosyl fluorides as glycosyl donors and allow they allow the preparation of a myriad of carbohydrate derivatives.

The 1,2-Migration Reaction

In the course of our investigations of the reactions of DAST with carbohydrate derivatives, we discovered that a 1,2-migration reaction occurs when carbohydrates, which have an unprotected 2-hydroxy group trans to the anomeric substituent, such as (44) (Figure 9), are treated with DAST (16). We later learned that Hasegawa et al. concurrently reported the 1,2-migration reaction in α-L-talofuranoside derivatives (17).

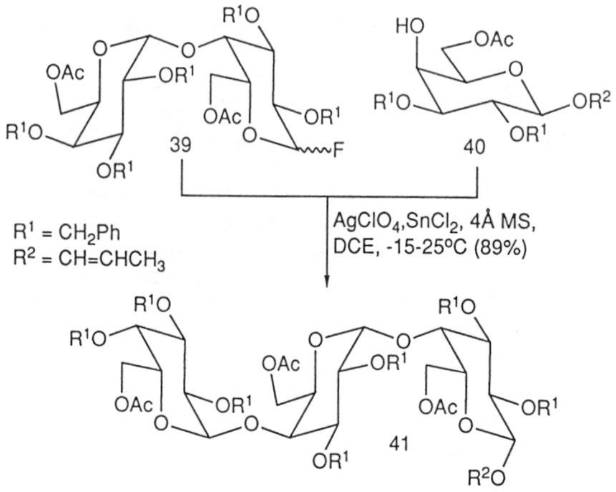

Figure 7.   Synthesis of α(1→4) Galactosides.

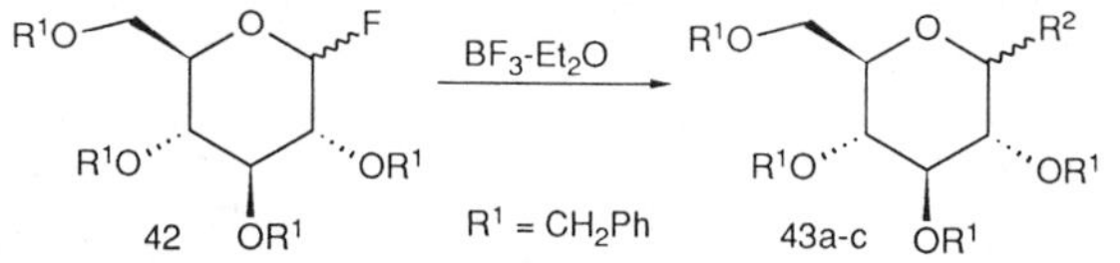

Entry	Conditions	Product	Yield (α:β)
1	TMSCN, CH$_2$Cl$_2$, 0°C	43a R^2 = CN	90% (3:1)
2	TMSN$_3$, CH$_2$Cl$_2$, 0-25°C	43b R^2 = N$_3$	90% (10:1)
3	(R^{1}O)$_2$P(O)OSnBu$_3$, Et$_2$O, 0-25°	43c R^2 = O(O)P(OR^1)$_2$	50% (10:1)

Figure 8.   Boron Trifluoride-Etherate as a Glycosidation Promoter.

This reaction may occur by one or both of the mechanisms shown in Figure 9. It appears that the DAST reagent first reacts with the 2-hydroxyl group of the carbohydrate derivative (46) to form a diethylaminosulfur difluoride species (47). Elimination then occurs to form either the "onium" (48) or oxonium (49) intermediates. The "onium" intermediate (48) seems plausible only in the case of the thioglycosides (X=SR). Although the anti product is often exclusively formed, in some cases anomeric mixtures of glycosyl fluorides are obtained; however, in every case studied, the 1,2-migration products contained the migrated moiety on the same face of the ring on which they originated. These findings suggest the intermediacy of the oxonium intermediate (49). The coupling reactions of glycosyl fluorides presented earlier allow the conversion of the 1,2-migration products into a variety of useful carbohydrate derivatives.

A variety of anomeric substituents undergo this novel migration reaction; indeed, not only could common hydroxyl protecting groups, such as -OMe, -OAc, and -OCH$_2$Ph, be induced to undergo this migration, but also O-sugar and other more complex substituents. The migration of the 1-O-substituents essentially results in the inversion of configuration at C-2. When phenyl thioglycosides undergo the 1,2-migration reaction, (2-phenylthio)glycosyl fluorides are obtained, which we have shown to be useful intermediates for the synthesis of 2-deoxy glycosides.

Synthesis of 2-Deoxy Glycosides

We envisioned that by coupling (2-phenylthio)glycosyl fluorides with glycosyl acceptors followed by removal of the 2-phenylthio moiety, 2-deoxy glycosides may be prepared (16). Moreover, it was anticipated that the 2-phenylthio group may be utilized to influence the anomeric selectivity of the glycosidation reaction. We reasoned that, by treating a phenyl β-thioglucoside with DAST, the corresponding (2-phenylthio)mannosyl fluoride may be obtained in which the phenylthio moiety would remain on the β-face of the carbohydrate ring; accordingly, by treatment of a phenyl α-thiomannoside with DAST, the corresponding (2-phenylthio)glucosyl fluoride would be obtained in which the phenylthio moiety would remain on the α-face of the carbohydrate ring. If the 2-phenylthio group could be induced to influence the glycosidation reaction, (2-phenylthio)-α- and β-glycosides may be able to be selectively formed from the (2-phenylthio)mannosyl and (2-phenylthio)glucosyl fluorides, respectively. Upon desulfurization, the desired 2-deoxy-α- and β-glycosides would be obtained. In order to realize this scenario, the required intermediates of the gluco- and manno- configuration were prepared with both of the intermediates protected in the same manner to expedite analysis of the products obtained.

In attempts to couple the (2-phenylthio)glycosyl fluorides with a glycosyl acceptor (methyl 2,3,4-tri-O-acetyl-α-D-glucoside, 53, Figure 10) many promoters, solvents and reaction conditions were surveyed. Most of the Lewis acid promoters that were investigated gave low yields of the corresponding glycosides, but tin(II) chloride was found to be a highly effective promoter of the glycosidation reaction. We found that the reaction of the (2-phenylthio)mannosyl fluoride (51) with the glycosyl acceptor (53) in dichloromethane with

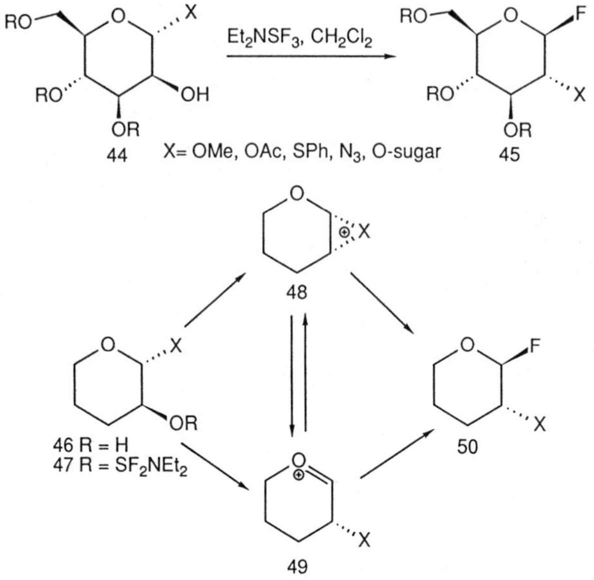

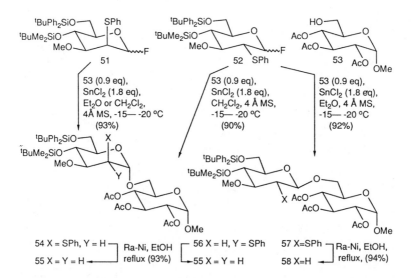

Figure 9.   The 1,2-Migration Reaction.(Adapted from Ref. 16.)

Figure 10.   Synthesis of 2-Deoxy Glycosides.(Adapted from Ref. 16.)

tin(II) chloride as the promoter in the presence of 4A molecular sieves at -15–20°C, provided the (2-phenylthio)-α-mannoside (54), exclusively, in 91% yield. Also, when the reaction was carried out in ether, under the same conditions, the α-glycoside was again stereospecifically obtained in 93% yield. It was expected that the α-glycoside would be selectively obtained due to the influence of the axial 2-phenylthio moiety and the anomeric effect (8). Desulfurization of the glycoside was efficiently accomplished with Raney nickel in refluxing ethanol to afford the 2-deoxy-α-glycoside (55) in 93% yield.

We first attempted to form the (2-phenylthio)-β-glucoside from glycosyl donor (52) and glycosyl acceptor (53), utilizing dichloromethane as the solvent, with similar conditions as for the previous example; however, the (2-phenylthio)-α-glucoside (56) was predominantly obtained (α:β ratio = 10:1). Nevertheless, it was pleasing to discover that when the reaction was carried out in ether, under otherwise the same conditions, the (2-phenylthio)-β-glucoside (57) was selectively formed (α:β ratio = 1:16) in 92% yield. This glycoside was desulfurized with Raney nickel to provide the 2-deoxy-β-glycoside (58) in 94% yield. Of course, we expected to achieve the selective formation of the β-glycoside in this glycosidation reaction, due to the participation of the equatorial 2-phenylthio moiety; however, it was surprising that the β-glycoside was not selectively obtained when the reaction was carried out in dichloromethane. We felt that the ability of the 2-phenylthio moiety to influence the glycosidation reaction was dependent on a solvent/promoter interaction, although the effect of the polarity of the solvent was also considered.

Utilizing the empirical results of the glycosidation reactions and the information obtained in a solvent effect study, we developed plausible mechanisms for the glycosidation reactions of the (2-phenylthio)glycosyl fluorides. As previously stated, it was expected that the (2-phenylthio)mannosyl fluoride (51, Figure 11), which contains the 2-phenylthio moiety in the axial orientation, would selectively provide the α-glycoside (61). This product presumably could be formed either by the nucleophilic opening of the episulphonium ion (59) or by the reaction of the intermediate oxonium ion (60), due to the anomeric effect (8); indeed, the α-glycoside was exclusively obtained when either dichloromethane or ether was used as the solvent. However, in attempts to form the β-glycoside from the (2-phenylthio)glucosyl fluoride (52, Figure 12), a significant solvent effect was found to exist.

We perceive that this solvent effect is due to the competition between the equatorial phenylthio moiety and the solvent for the active sites of the promoter, tin(II) chloride. When ether is employed as the solvent, it may form a complex with the active sites of the promoter (62 and 63), thereby allowing the participation of the sulfur and the formation of the episulphonium intermediate (64). Reaction of the glycosyl acceptor with this transient intermediate selectively forms the β-glycoside (65). We found that when the reaction was carried out in dichloromethane, in the presence of dimethyl sulfide, the β-glycoside was obtained, presumably due to the complexation of the additive to the active sites of the promoter. When dichloromethane is used as the solvent with no dimethyl sulfide

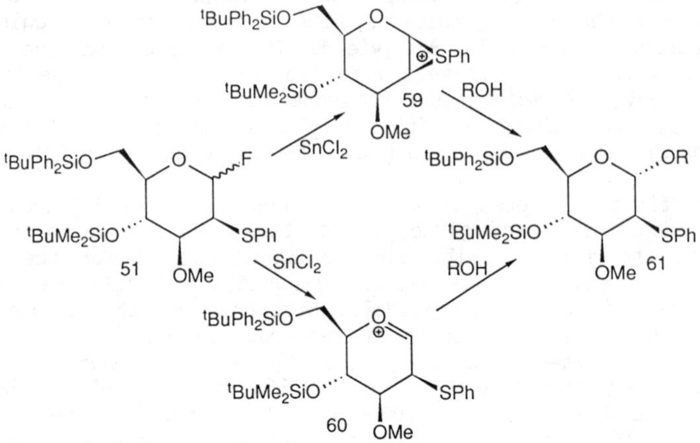

Figure 11. Mechanism for the Formation of (2-Phenylthio)-α-Glyco-
sides.

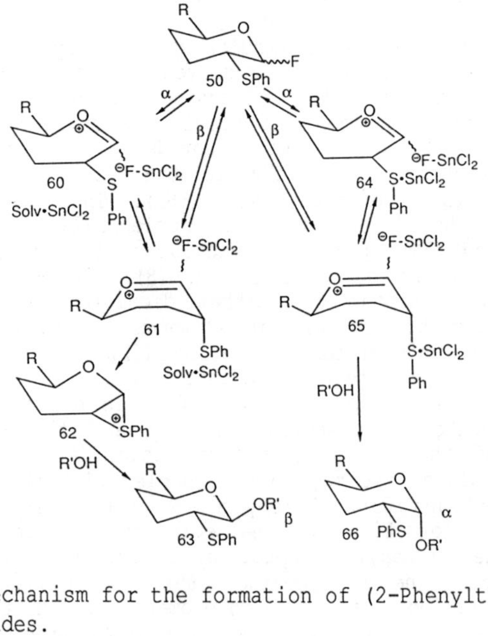

Figure 12. Mechanism for the formation of (2-Phenylthio)-β-Glyco-
sides.

added,the promoter engages the sulfur (66 and 67), thus preventing its participation, and the α-glycoside is predominantly formed via the oxonium ion (67), due to the influence of the anomeric effect (8). Indeed, it is interesting to note that either the α- or β-glycoside can both be selectively formed from the same glycosyl donor merely by changing the reaction solvent.

Future Perspectives

The use of glycosyl fluorides as glycosyl donors should continue to find applications in the area of carbohydrate chemistry. Although many methods exist for the formation of glycosyl fluorides and their use in the formation of the glycosidic linkage, the search for more efficient methods will continue. The investigation of new reagents for promoting the reactions of glycosyl fluorides should be particularly active. The untapped potential of the 1,2-migration reaction will allow novel approaches to 2-deoxy glycosides and other permutations of the glycosidic linkage. Additional mechanistic studies would greatly advance the understanding of the reactions of glycosyl fluorides and may provide the key to the development of new methodologies.

Acknowledgments

The authors would like to thank the members of the Nicolaou group who contributed to these investigations.

Literature Cited

1. Penglis, A. A. E. Adv. Carbohydr. Chem. Biochem. 1981, 38, 195.
2. Card, P. J. J. Carbohydr. Chem. 1985, 4, 451.
3. Nicolaou, K. C.; Dolle, R. E.; Papahatjis, D. P.; Randall, J. L. J. Am. Chem. Soc. 1984, 106, 4189.
4. Mukaiyama, T.; Murai, Y.; Shoda, S. Chem. Lett. 1981, 431.
5. Nicolaou, K. C.; Randall, J. L.; Furst, G. T. ibid. 1985, 107, 5556.
6. Sadozai, K. K.; Nukada, T.; Ito, Y.; Nakahara, Y.; Ogawa, T.; Kobata, A. Carbohydr. Res. 1986, 157, 101
7. Nakahara, Y.; Ogawa, T. Tetrahedron Lett. 1987, 28, 2731.
8. Lemieux, R. U.; Hendriks, K. B.; Stick, R. V.; James, K. J. Am. Chem. Soc. 1975, 97, 4056.
9. Paulsen, H. Angew. Chem. Int. Ed. Engl. 1982, 21, 155.
10. a) Dolle, R. E.; Nicolaou, K. C. J. Am. Chem. Soc. 1985, 107, 1691; b) Dolle, R. E.; Nicolaou, K. C. ibid. 1985, 107, 1695.
11. Sato, S.; Ito, T.; Ogawa, T. Carbohydr. Res. 1986, 155, C1.
12. Koike, K.; Sugimoto, M.; Sato, S.; Ito, Y.; Nakahara,Y.; Ogawa, T. ibid. 1987, 163, 189.
13. Lemieux, R. U.; Koto, S. Tetrahedron 1974, 30, 1933.
14. a) Nicolaou, K. C.; Chucholowski, A.; Dolle, R. E.; Randall, J. L. J. Chem. Soc. Chem. Comm. 1984, 1155; b) Nicolaou, K. C.;Dolle, R. E.; Chucholowski, A.; Randall, J. L. ibid. 1984, 1156.
15. a) Araki, Y.; Watanabe, Kuan, F-H.; Itoh, K.; Kobayashi, N. Carbohydr. Res. 1984, 127, C5; b) Kunz, H.; Sager, W. Helv.

Chem. Acta. 1985, 68, 283; c) Araki, Y.; Kobayashi, N.;
Watanabe, K.; Ishido, Y. J. Carbohydr. Chem. 1985, 4, 565
16. Nicolaou, K. C.; Ladduwahetty, T.; Randall, J. L.; Chucholowski,
A. J. Am. Chem. Soc. 1986, 108, 2466.
17. Hasegawa, A.; Goto, M.; Kiso, M. J. Carbohydr. Chem. 1985, 4,
627.

RECEIVED January 15, 1988

Chapter 3

Chemoenzymatic Synthesis of Fluorosugars

C.-H. Wong, D. G. Dreckhammer, and H. M. Sweers

Departments of Chemistry and of Biochemistry and Biophysics, Texas A&M University, College Station, TX 77843

Several practical enzymatic procedures have been developed for the synthesis of fluorocarbohydrates. The enzymes fructose-1,6-diphosphate aldolase and glucose isomerase are used in the synthesis of 6-deoxy-6-fluorohexoses. Hexokinase is used for the preparation of a number of fluorohexose-6-phosphates, two of them are further converted to 2-deoxy-2-fluoropentose-5 phosphates. When ATP is required, it is regenerated from ADP catalyzed by pyruvate kinase in the presence of phosphoenol pyruvate. Lipases are used as catalysts in selective deprotection of peracylated sugars, the products of which are converted to fluorosugars by reaction with diethylaminosulfur trifluoride. Incorporation of F into oligosaccharide is illustrated by a gram-scale synthesis of 6'-deoxy-6'-fluorosucrose catalyzed by sucrose synthetase coupled with enzymatic regenerations of UDP, UTP and UDP-glucose.

Fluorinated Sugars in which one of the hydroxyl groups is replaced with the fluorine group can be strong inhibitors of the nonfluorinated species in biochemical processes and are of interest as potential pharmaceuticals or pharmacological probes (1-4). The inhibitions are mainly due to the difference of C-F and C-OH in reactivity and the similarity of both groups in polarity and bond length. Examples have been shown in which fluorinated monosaccharides inhibit the glycosylation of glycoproteins. 6-Fluoro-L-fucose (5), 6-deoxy-6-fluoro-galactose (5), 4-deoxy-4-fluoromannose (6), and 2-deoxy-2-fluoromannnose have been shown to inhibit the

0097–6156/88/0374–0029$06.00/0
○ 1988 American Chemical Society

incorporation of the corresponding nonfluorinated sugars
into glycoproteins. Mechanistic studies on the
glycosylation of some viral glycoproteins have indicated
that the fluorosugars are converted into the
corresponding nucleoside diphosphates which inhibit the
assembly of the lipid-linked oligosaccharides catalyzed
by the appropriate glycosyl transferases (5-8). The
synthesis of fluorocarbohydrates currently depends on
chemical procedures (9-14) which very often require
multiple protection and deprotection steps to overcome
the problems of stereoselectivity. Recent research has
been focused on the development of milder and more
selective methods for the incorporation of fluorine into
carbohydrates. This review is only focused on the recent
developments in the enzymatic approach to the synthesis
of fluorinated carbohydrates.
The approach has the advantages that the reactions are
catalytic, stereoselective and that they are carried out
under mild conditions in aqueous solution, with minimum
protection of the fuuncional groups.

Aldolase/Isomerase-Catalyzed Reactions

We have developed preparative enzymatic syntheses of
several unusual hexoketoses using fructose-1,6-
diphosphate aldolase (FDP-aldolase, E.C.4.1.2.13) as
catalyst and dihydroxyacetone phosphate (DHAP) and an
aldehyde as substrates (15). The enzyme appears to be
very specific for DHAP but will accept a variety of
aldehydes as acceptors. The ketose-1-phosphates prepared
are converted to the phosphate free ketoses after removal
of the phosphate group by acid- or phosphatase-catalyzed
hydrolysis. The ketoses can be isomerized
stereospecifically to aldoses catalyzed by glucose
isomerase (E.C.5.3.1.5.) from _Flavobacteriuum
arborescens_. The equilibrium mixtures of aldoses and
ketoses are then separated by chromatography on Dowex 50
(Ba^{++}) or Dowex 1 (HSO_3^-). Figure 1 illustrates the
preparation of a mixture of 6-deoxy-6-fluoro-D-fructose
(5) and 6-deoxy-6-fluoro-L-sorbose (6), the former is
selectively isomerized to 6-deoxy-6-fluoro-D-glucose (7)
in the presence of glucose isomerase. The equilibrium
mixture of (5) and (7) contains 80% of (7). Detailed
procedures for these preparations were reported (15).
The substrate dihydroxyacetone phosphate (DHAP) can be
prepared enzymatically (15) or chemically (15,16).
Alternatively, it can be replaced with a mixture of
dihydroxyacetone and a small amount of inorganic
arsenate. The proposed mechanism for this interesting
process is shown in Figure 2. In solution,
dihydroxyacetone reversibly reacts with arsenate to form
dihydroxyacetone arsenate which is analogous to DHAP and
thus accepted by the enzyme as a substrate. The arsenate
moiety of the aldol product is then dissociated

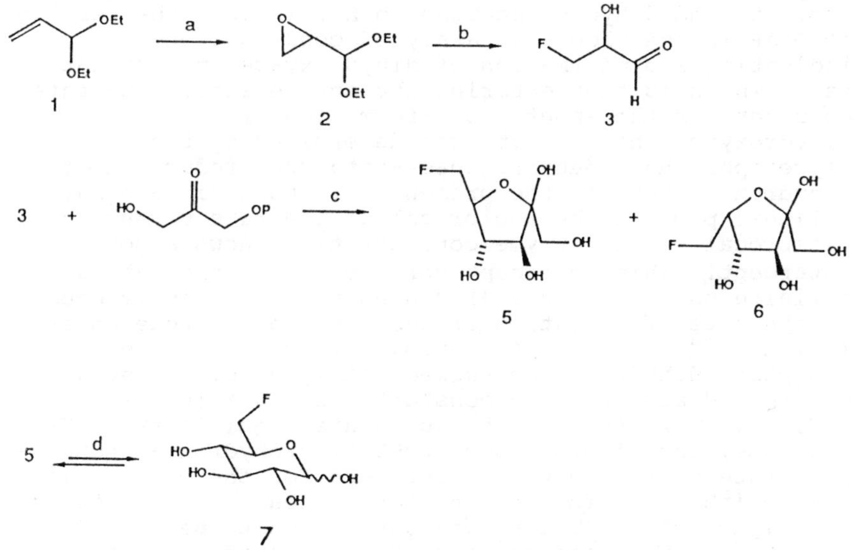

Figure 1.   Preparation of fluorosugars via enzymatic aldol reactions. a) C_6H_5CN/H_2O_2. b) 1, KHF_2, H^+. c) 1, FDP-aldolase; 2, H^+. d)   glucose isomerase.

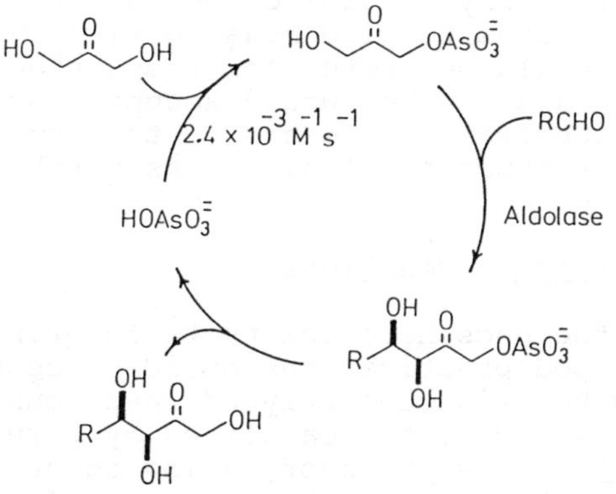

Figure 2.   Use of dihydroxyacetone and arsenate as substrate in FDP-aldolase reactions.   The rate constant was determined in Figure 3.

spontaneously and used repeatedly. The evidence which
supports this mechanism is the following. Both inorganic
arsenate and dihydroxyacetone do not inhibit the reaction
of DHAP in the aldolase-catalyzed condensations,
indicating a preformation of dihydroxyacetone arsenate
ester which is then entering the active site. The rate
constant for the spontaneous formation of
dihydroxyacetone arsenate was determined by the
glycerophosphate dehydrogenase-catalyzed reduction of
dihydroxyacetone in the presence of inorganic arsenate.
A linear plot of the reciprocal of the rate versus the
reciprocal of the enzyme concentration shows a non-zero
intercept. This intercept corresponds to the rate at
infinite enzyme (Figure 3) concentration which is equal
to the rate of formation of the dihydroxyacetone ester
(2.4×10^{-3} M^{-1} s^{-1}). A previous study on glucose-6-
phosphate dehydrogenase showed that glucose-6-arsenate
was formed and the rate constant was 6.3×10^{-6} $M^{-1}s^{-1}$
(17). In our study on the substrate specificity of FDP
aldolase, the compound 3-deoxy-3-fluorohydroxyacetone-1-
phosphate was found not a substrate for the enzyme; it
was an inhibitor for the enzymatic cleavage of fructose-
1,6-diphosphate. The k_i was determined to be 3 mM
(Figure 4). When sodium borohydride was added to the
mixture of aldolase and 3-deoxy-3-fluorohydroxyacetone-1-
phosphate, no inactivation of aldolase was observed,
indicating that a Schiff base is not formed. The Schiff
base intermediate in the mixture of DHAP and aldolase has
previously been trapped by reduction with sodium
borohydride to inactivate the enzyme (8). The inhibitor
may be useful for study of the active site of the enzyme.
        There have been more than 10 different aldolases
isolated; they catalyze aldol condensations using
different substrates to give sugar derivatives (19).
These enzymes would be useful for the synthesis of
fluorinated sugars if they would accept fluorinated
molecules as substrates. We are in the process of
exploring other types of aldolases as synthetic
catalysts.

Hexokinase-Catalyzed Reactions

To introduce the phosphate moiety to fluorinated sugars,
we have developed practical enzymatic procedures based on
ATP-requiring hexokinase-catalyzed reactions coupled with
an ATP regeneration system catalyzed by pyruvate kinase
(Figure 5) (20). The phosphorylating agent
phosphoenolpyruvate used in the regeneration of ATP can
be easily prepared based on the improved procedure in
which the monopotassium salt of phosphoenolpyruvate was
obtained as crystals (21). The relative activities of
hexokinase on fluorinated hexoses are shown in Figure 5.
Both yeast hexokinase and pyruvate kinase are quite
stable in the immobilized forms (20). Phosphoenol

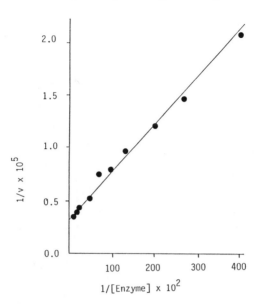

Figure 3. Reciprocal of the rate (M/min) of glycerophosphate dehydrogenase-catalyzed reduction of dihydroxyacetone in the presence of 5 mM arsenate vs the reciprocal of enzyme concentration (mg/mL). Reactions were carried out in Tris buffer (20 mM, pH 8.0) containing NADH (0.1 mM), dihydroxyacetone (50 mM), glycerophosphate dehydrogenase and sodium arsenate (5 mM). The decrease in absorbance at 340 nm was monitored versus time.

pyruvate is a strong phosphorylating agent and is quite stable in solution (ΔG^{o} for hydrolysis = 16 kcal/mol, t1/2 at PH 7 = 30 days) (19). This allows us to synthesize fluorinated hexose-6-phosphates on gram scales without difficulty although some fluorosugars are weak substrates for hexokinase. Of the fluorohexose phosphates prepared, two of them have been converted to 2-deoxy-2-fluoropentose-5-phosphates. The detailed reactions are shown in Figure 6. The phosphate moiety not only serves as a protecting group in the transformation of hexose phosphate to pentose phosphate, it also locks the pentose phosphates in the furanose form which is desired in the synthesis of nucleoside monophosphates.

Lipase-Catalyzed Deprotection of Acylated Sugars

Selective deprotection of peracylated sugars is of interest in carbohydrate chemistry. The free OH group of the deprotected sugar can be converted to the F group by

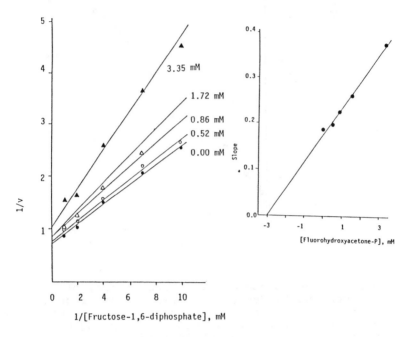

Figure 4.   Reciprocal plots of aldolase activity at
different concentrations of 3-deoxy-3-
fluorohydroxyacetone-1-phosphate.   The reaction was
coupled with glycerophosphate dehydrogenase in the
presence of NADH to determine the enzyme activity.
(see ref. 15).   Inserted, slope of the reciprocal
plots of aldolase activity vs 3-deoxy-3-fluoro-
hydroxyacetone-1-phosphate.

reaction with diethylaminosulfurtrifluoride (DAST) (22).
Of the different acylated sugars tested, an acyl group
with a longer chain is a better substrate than that with
shorter chain and the primary position is selectively
hydrolyzed (22).   In a typical 100-mmol scale reaction,
the tetrapentanoyl derivative of α-methyl D-
glucopyranoside was selectively hydrolyzed by the lipase
from Candida cylindraceae to the 6-OH derivative in >90%
yield.   Similar selectivity was observed in the
hydrolysis of the other acyl derivatives of α- and β-
methyl D-hexopyranosides including galactose, mannose, N-
acetylglucosamine and N-acetylmannosamine. (22)   These 6-
OH sugar derivatives can be used for synthesis of 6-F
hexoses by reaction with DAST.   Table I indicates
relative and specific activities of Candida lipase-
catalyzed hydrolysis of different sugar esters at C-6
position.   All the products were isolated by silica gel

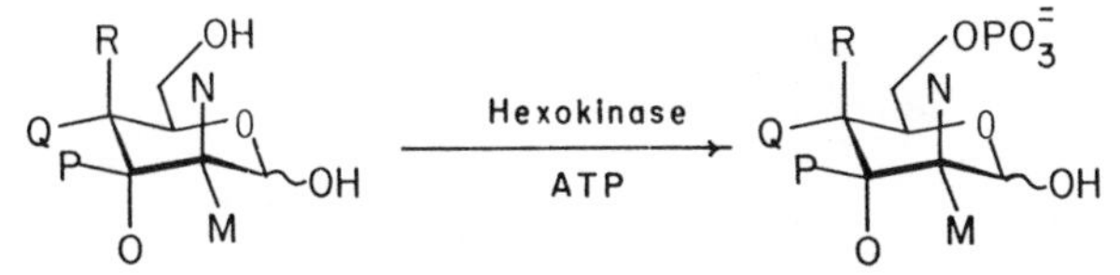

Cmpd	M	N	O	P	Q	R	X	Km (mM)	Vmax (Umg⁻¹)
a	OH	H	H	OH	OH	H	O	0.17	300
b	F			•				0.19	150
c	H	F						0.41	260
d	F	F						0.13	160
e			F	H				82	30
f				F				70	30
g					F			84	30
h						H	F	–	3

Figure 5. Hexokinase-catalyzed phosphorylation of fluorinated hexoses coupled with an ATP regeneration system using phosphoenol pyruvate as phosphorylating agent and pyruvate kinase as catalyst.

column chromatography eluted with $CHCl_3$: MeOH (10:1) and the structures proven by microanalysis and ^{13}C-NMR analysis using the deuterium induced shifts (DIS) technique (24). The addition of dimethylformamide (10%) to the candida lipase-catalyzed hydrolysis of glucose pentaacetate changes the regioselectivity. In reaction with glucose pentaacetate, 1,2,3-tri-O-acetyl-α-D-glucose and 1,2,3,4-tetra-O-acetyl-β-D-glucose were isolated in 73% and 27% yield respectively. The structures of the compounds are shown in Table III. All shifts are in ppm from TMS. The DIS numbers are in parentheses. Negative values indicate upfield shifts. Both compounds were identified by using the DIS techniques (Table II). They show expected upfield shift of the deacylated carbon. When the peracetylated sugars were hydrolyzed by porcine pancreas lipase in the presence or absence of 10% DMF, the same regio selectivity was observed, all being hydrolyzed at C-1 position preferentially (Table III). The products were isolated by extraction with ethyl

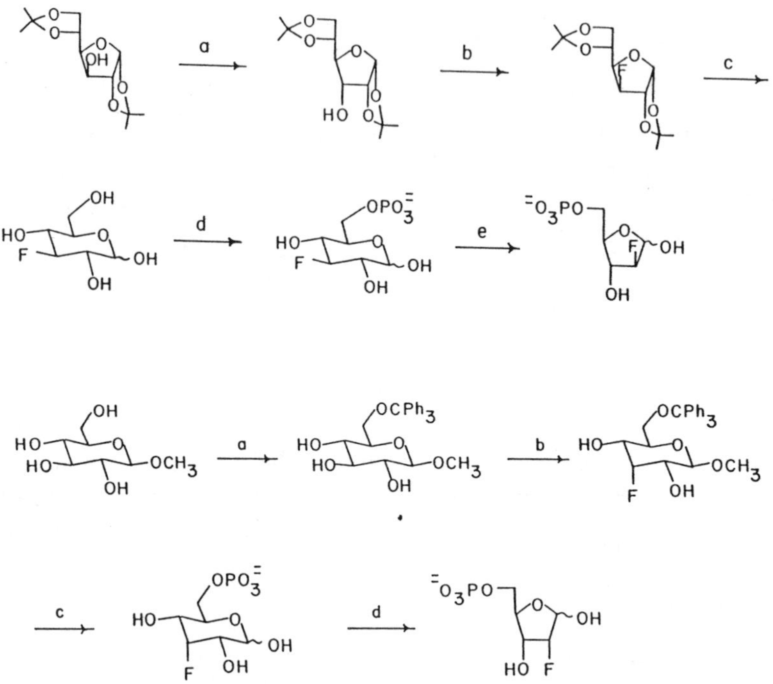

Figure 6.   Preparation of 2-deoxy-2-fluoro-arabinose-
5-phosphate (upper scheme) and 2-deoxy-2-D-ribose-5-
phosphate (lower scheme).   Upper scheme: a) 1,
pyridium dichromate. 2, $NaBH_4$/70% aq. ethanol, 92%
yield.   b) DAST/CH_2Cl_2/pyridine, 88 % yield.   c)
Dowex 50 (H+)/H_2O, 92% Yield.   d)
ATP/hexokinase/phosphoenol pyruvate/pyruvate kinase,
90% yield. e) Pb(OAc)$_4$/H$^+$, 64% yield.   Lower scheme:
a) Ph_3CCl/pyridine, 70 % yield.   b) DAST/CH_2Cl_2, 50%
yield.   c) 1.80% AcOH/Dowex 50 (H$^+$); 2.
ATP/hexokinase system as above, 90% yield.   d)
Pb(OAc)$_4$/H$^+$, 60 % yield.

Table I. Lipase-Catalyzed Selective Hydrolysis of Different Sugar Esters at C-6 position

Substrate	Specific Activity[a]	Relative Activity
Me α-D-glucopyranoside, tetrapentanoate	0.020	0.13
Me α-D-glucopyranoside, tetraoctanoate	0.153	1.00
Me β-D-glucopyranoside, tetraoctanoate	0.044	0.29
Me α-D-galactopyranoside, tetrapentanoate	0.017	0.11
Me α-D-mannopyranoside, tetrapentanoate	0.015	0.10
α D-glucose, pentaacetate	0.00	0.00
	0.04b	0.26b
β-D-glucose, pentaacetate	<0.001c	<0.01c
Me N-Acetylglucosamine, tripentanoate	0.02	0.13
Me N-acetylmanosamine, tripentanoate	0.01	0.13

[a]The enzyme was from <u>Candida cylindracea</u>. Specific activity = 1 U/mg protein. 1 U = 1 μmol of acid released per min. All reactions were carried out in 100 mL of 0.1 M sodium phosphate buffer, pH 7, containing 0.2 M NaCl, 3 mM $CaCl_2$, the substrate (1 g in 5 mL of acetone was added), and the enzyme (0.1 g). The mixture was stirred at room temperature and the pH was automatically controlled by adding 0.02 N NaOH until one equivalent of base was consumed (2-3 days). The mixture was then extracted with chloroform to isolate the products. Regioselectivity of each reaction was > 95% unless otherwise mentioned.
[b]The reaction was carried out in 0.05 M sodium phosphate, pH 7, containing 10% DMF until the substrate disappeared. The same amount of enzyme as substrate by weight was used. The isolated products contain 76% of the corresponding 4,6-di-OH product and 22% of the 6-OH product. In the absence of DMF, C-1 was hydrolyzed to the 1-OH species in 50% isolated yield. In 0.1M phosphate, however, no reaction was observed.
[c]Under the same condition as b, the 4, 6-di-OH species was the major product (51%) in a 3-day reaction. Other products were unidentified.

Table II.   ^{13}C-Shifts of DIS Experiments on Candida Lipase-Catalyzed Hydrolysis of α-glucose pentaacetate[a]

Compound	C1	C2	C3	C4	C5	C6
α-D-glucose 1,2,3,4-tetraacetate	88.67 (+0.02)	68.95 (+0.01)	69.28 (+0.02)	67.82 (+0.01)	71.71 (0.00)	60.23 (0.13)
α-D-glucose 1,2,3-triacetate	89.03 (+0.03)	69.19 (+0.02)	71.85 (-0.03)	67.88 (-0.19)	73.67 (+4.04)	60.83 (-0.19)

[a]All shifts are indicated in ppm from TMS. The deuterium induced shift numbers are in parenthesis upon exchange with D_2O. Negative values indicate upfield shifts.

Table III. Selective Hydrolysis of Peracetylated Sugars at the C-1 Position by Porcine Pancreatic Lipase Catalysis[a]

Substrate	Product	Regioselectivity*/ Isolated yield	α/β ratio
		>90	>50
		>90	>50
		>90	3
		>90	3
		>90	11

[a]All reactions (1g substrate/100 mL/g enzyme) were carried out at room temperature in sodium phosphate buffer (0.05M, pH 7.0). During the reaction, the pH was maintained by the addition of 0.05N NaOH until 1 equivalent of base was consumed. The product was isolated by extraction with ethylacetate and purified by flash chromotography on silica gel using ethyl acetate/petroleum ether as the mobile phase.
*Determined by comparing the indicated product to other byproducts based on the GC analysis of the silylated derivatives.

acetate and purified by flash chromatography on silica
gel eluted with ethyl acetate/petroleum ether and
characterized by ^{13}C-NMR (Table IV).
The structures of the compounds are shown in Table III.
All shifts are in ppm from TMS. The DIS numbers are in
parentheses. Negative
values indicate upfield shifts.

Fluorinated Di- and Oligosaccharides

The fluorinated monosaccharides can be incorporated into
disaccharides and oligosaccharides. For example, 6'-
deoxy-6'-fluorosucrose and 4'-deoxy-4'-fluorosucrose were
prepared by reaction of UDP-glucose with the fluorinated
fructose derivative catalyzed by sucrose synthetase (25).
Based on the synthetic strategy we have developed (Figure
7) (26), the synthesis of di- and oligosaccharides can be
scaled up if the cofactors (e.g. UDP, UTP and UDP-sugar)
are regenerated in the reactions. Indeed, the process
has been shown to be quite practical for synthesis of
oligosaccharides on 50-g
scales. To illustrate the feasibility of this
multienzyme system in preparative synthesis of
fluorinated oligosaccharide, we have carried
out the synthesis of 6'-deoxy-6'-
fluorosucrose, a potent ligand for sucrose carrier
protein (25), on 5-g scale (Figure 7). This synthetic
scheme involves coimmobilization of four enzymes in
polyacrylamide gel (19) and renegeration of the cofactors
UTP, UDP, and UDP-glucose. At the conclusion of the
reaction, all the
enzymes were recovered with > 80% retention of activity.

Table IV. ^{13}C-Shifts of DIS Experiments on Porcine
Pancreas Lipase-Catalyzed Hydrolysis of Peracetylated
Sugars

Compound		C1	C2	C3	C4	C5	C6
1		91.60	52.58	68.70	67.45	71.30	62.49
		(-0.12)	(-0.05)	(+0.04)	(-0.01)	(-0.01)	(0.00)
2		93.51	51.44	66.53	67.90	69.56	63.09)
		(-0.12)	(-0.04)	(-0.04)	(-0.01)	(+0.08)	(-0.03)
3	α	90.12	68.84	70.21	67.22	71.43	62.29
		(-0.13)	(+0.02)	(+0.03)	(0.00)	(0.00)	(+0.03)
3	β	95.48	72.18	72.74	68.74	73.21	62.29
		(-0.13)	(-0.01)	(+0.05)	(+0.02)	(-0.01)	(+0.03)
4	α	90.72	68.48	67.55	66.14	68.70	60.66
		(-0.14)	(+0.01)	(-0.03)	(-0.03)	(-0.01)	(+0.03)
4	β	96.02	67.46	70.98	70.85	71.07	60.66
		(-0.14)	(+0.01)	(-0.08)	(-0.05)	(-0.02)	(+0.03)
5		92.23	69.20	68.42	66.46	70.52	62.87
		(-0/02)	(+0.07)	(-0.04)	(0.00)	(+0.01)	(+0.01)

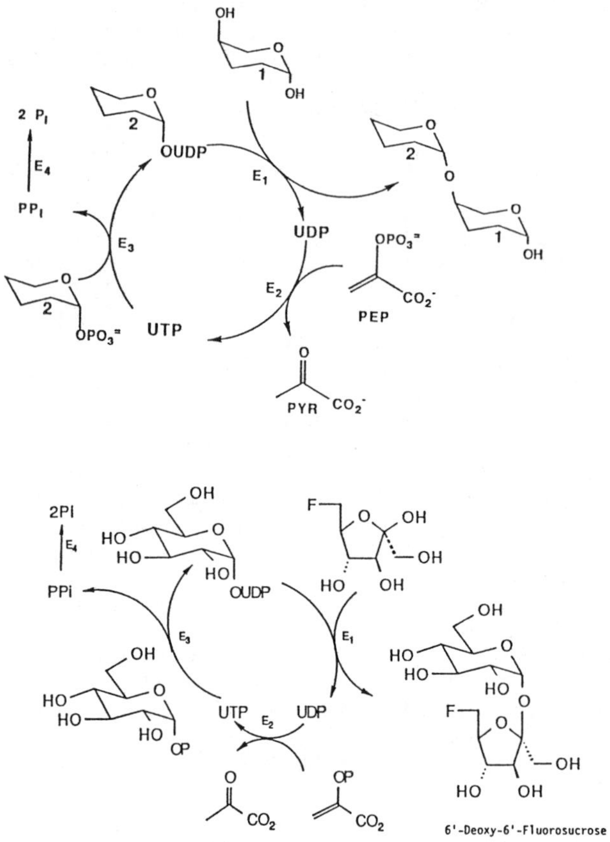

Figure 7.   Strategy for oligosaccharide synthesis.
E1:   glycosyl transferase.   E2:   pyruvate kinase.
E3:   UDP-sugar phosphorylase.   E4:   pyrophosphatase.
(Below)   Synthesis of 6'-deoxy-6'-fluorosucrose.   El,
sucrose synthetase; E2, pyruvate kinase; E3, UDP-
glucose pyrophosphorylase; E4, pyrophosphatase.   All
enzymes (150 U each) are co-immobilized in
polyacrylamide gel.   The reactions are carried out in
triethanolamine buffer (50 mM) containing $MgCl_2$ (10
mM) with pH being controlled at 7.5 by addition of 1N
NaOH.   The 500-mL reaction mixture contains glucose-
1-phosphate (8 mmol), phosphoenolpyruvate (10 mmol)
and UDP (0.2 mmol) was stirred at 25 °C for 24 h.
The product was isolated by Bio-gel P-2
chromatography as described before for the synthesis
of lactosamine (26) to give the product (2.1 g).

CONCLUSION

Several enzymatic methods in conjunction with conventional organic methods provide new synthetic routes to fluorinated sugars. These new methods allow preparative synthesis of sugars containing the fluorine probe for use in the NMR study of receptor-substrate interactions of enzymes, of cell-surface glycoproteins, and of other systems related to biochemical recognition (27). Similar procedures could be used for the efficient synthesis of ^{18}F-labeled sugars which are useful as tracers (28). The combined chemical/enzymatic approach also provides new routes to a number of potentially useful antiviral and antibacterial fluorosugars and derivatives (29,30).

Acknowledgments
Support of this work by the National Science Foundation (CHE 8318217 and the Presidential Young Investigator program) is gratefully acknowledged.

Literature Cited

1. Taylor, N.F.in Ciba Fdn. Symp: Carbon-Fluorine Compounds. Elsevier and Associated Scientific Publishers, Amsterdam, 1972, 212-38.
2. Biochemistry involving Carbon-Fluorine Bonds: Filler, R., Ed.; ACS Symposium Series, American Chemical Society, Washington D.C., 1976.
3. Walsh, C. Adv. Enzymol. 1983, 54, 197-289.
4. Sharpe, A.G.,in Ciba Found. Symp:Carbon-Fluorine Compounds. Elsevier, Amsterdam 1972, 33-54.
5. Sufrin, J.R.; Bernacki, R.J.; Morin, M.J.; Korytnyk, W. J. Med. Chem. 1980, 23, 143-9.
6. Grier, T.J.; Rasmussen, J.R. J. Biol.Chem. 1984, 259 1027-30.
7. McDowell, W.; Datema, R.; Romero, P.A.; Schwarz, R.T. Biochemistry, 1985, 24 8145-57.
8. Card, P.J. J. Carbohydr. Chem. 1985, 4, 451-87.
9. Kent, P.W.in Ciba Found. Symp:Carbon-Fluorine Compounds, Elsevier, Amsterdam,1972, 169-213.
10. Penglis, A.A.E. Adv. Carbohydr. Chem. Biochem. 1981, 38, 195-285.
11. Foster, A.B.; Westwood, J.H. Carbohydrate Chemistry-VIth International Symposium on Carbohydrate Chemistry, 1972, p. 146-169.
12. Tewson, T.J. J. Org. Chem. 1983, 48, 3507-10.
13. Dessinges, A.; Olesker, A.; Lukacs, G. Carbohydrate Res. 1984, 126, c6.
14. Welch, J.T. Tetrahedron, 1987, 43, 3123-97.
15. Durrwachter, J.R.; Drueckhammer, D.G.; Nozaki, K.; Sweers, H.M.; Wong, C.-H. J. Am. Chem. Soc. 1986, 108, 7812-18.

16. Effenberger, F.; Straub, A. Tetrahedron Lett. 1987,
     28 1641-4.
17. Nour-Eldeen, A.F.; Craig, M.M.; Gresser, M.J. J.
     Biol. Chem. 1985. 260, 6836.
18. Grazi, E.; Cheng, T.; Horrecker, B.L. Biochem.
     Biophys. Res. Comm. 1962, 7, 250-6.
19. Whitesides, G.M.; Wong, C.-H. Angew, Chem. Int. Ed.
     1985. 24, 617-38.
20. Drueckhammer, D.G.; Wong, C.-H. J. Org. Chem. 1985,
     50, 5912-3.
21. Hirschbein, B.L.; Mazenod, F.P.; Whitesides, G.M. J
     Org. Chem. 1982, 47, 3766-8.
22. Sweers, H.M.; Wong, C.-H. J. Am. Chem.Soc. 1986,
     108, 5421-2.
23. Therisod, M.; Klibanov, A. J. Am. Chem. Soc. 1987,
     109, 3977-81.
24. Pfeffer, P.E.; Valentine, K.M.; Parrish, F.W. J. Am.
     Chem. Soc. 1979, 101, 1266-74.
25. Card, P.J.; Hitz, W.D.; Ripp, K.G. J. Am. Chem. Soc.
     1986, 108, 158-61.
26. Wong, C.-H.; Haynie, S.L.; Whitesides, G.M. J. Org.
     Chem. 1982, 47, 5416-8.
27. Dwek, R.A. in Ciba Found. Symp: Carbon-Fluorine
     Compounds. 1972, 239-79.
28. Ratib, O.; Phelps, M.; Huang, S.C.; Henze, E.;
     Selin, C.E., Shelbert, H.R. J. Nucl. Med. 1982, 23,
     577-82.
29. Schwarz, R.T.; Datema, R. Trends in Biochem. Sci.
     1980, 65-67.
30. Feizi, T.; Childs, R.A. Biochem. J. 1987,245, 1-11.

RECEIVED February 22, 1988

Chapter 4

Fluorinated Analogues of *myo*-Inositols as Biological Probes of Phosphatidylinositol Metabolism

James D. Moyer[1], Ofer Reizes[1], Nancy Malinowski[1], Cong Jiang[2], and David C. Baker[2]

[1]Laboratory of Biological Chemistry, Division of Cancer Treatment, National Cancer Institute, National Institutes of Health, Bethesda, MD 20892
[2]Department of Chemistry, University of Alabama, Tuscaloosa, AL 35487

Analogues of *myo*-inositol were synthesized wherein certain hydroxyl groups were replaced with fluorine, and these were examined as substrates for phosphatidylinositol (PI) synthetase. Fluorine substitution at the 2- and 4(6)-positions of *myo*-inositol (giving the *scyllo*- and *myo*-isomers, respectively) resulted in loss of any detectable substrate activity. Replacement of the hydroxyl at C-5 of *myo*-inositol resulted in retention of appreciable PI synthetase activity (ca. 26% for the equatorial 5-deoxy-5-fluoro-*myo*- and ca. 16% for the axially substituted 2-deoxy-2-fluoro-*neo*-inositol). These results are significant in that none of the eight diastereomers of *myo*-inositol are substrates for PI synthetase. Furthermore, it was shown that radiolabeled 5-deoxy-5-fluoro-*myo*-inositol is taken up by L1210 cells in a manner similar to that observed for *myo*-inositol. The analogue is incorporated into a lipid that is chromatographically similar to, but distinctly different from, PI. The lipid is hydrolyzed in base to a water-soluble form and is converted to the deoxyfluoro cyclitol upon treatment with phospholipase D.

Since *myo*-inositol (1) was first discovered by Scherer (1) in 1850 as a component of meat extract, the compound and its isomers and analogues, known collectively as cyclitols, have been the objects of intense study by both chemists and biochemists. During the first century following the discovery of *myo*-inositol (1), chemists, including Posternak, Angyal, and L. Anderson, devoted much effort to structure elucidation and synthesis of these compounds. By 1957 every diastereomer of *myo*-inositol (1) had been synthesized [cis-

0097–6156/88/0374–0043$06.00/0

myo-Inositol (1)

Inositol was the last to be definitively synthesized (2).], and
chemists had provided a vast array of derivatives and modified
cyclitols for study. Details of these developments are reviewed by
Posternak in his monograph (3), by Fletcher (4), by Angyal and L.
Anderson (5), and by L. Anderson (6) in their excellent surveys of
the field.

   myo-Inositol (1) was discovered as a constituent of
phospholipids in the tubercle bacilli by R. Anderson in 1930 (7),
and its presence in mammalian lipids was reported by Folch and
Woolley in 1942 (8). Folch pursued the work which resulted in the
identification of multiply phosphorylated myo-inositols (9-11) whose
presence in the phosphatidylinositol phosphates of mammals was
precisely determined by Brockerhoff and Ballou in 1961 (12).

   This body of chemical and biochemical work perhaps prompted
Posternak in his comprehensive treatise (3) to state

   "... the major problems in cyclitol chemistry are now
   solved. A good many organic and physical chemists will
   still be captivated by the beauty and clarity of cyclitol
   chemistry, but it is more than likely that it will be the
   numerous biological and biochemical questions that will
   attract most of the energy to be expended."

   While Posternak's prediction has proven to be accurate, it is
unlikely that he realized that there would be the intense interest
in inositol metabolism in the 1980's (13) that has resulted from the
recent discovery of the role of phosphatidylinositol in the action
of growth factors and hormones (reviewed in 14). This recent
discovery has also reawakened interest in cyclitols among medicinal
chemists as phosphatidylinositol is a key intermediate in the action
of a number of physiologically active biological compounds, a fact
which suggests new targets for drug design.

   The key to understanding the role of phosphoinositides in the
action of hormones and growth factors was the discovery that the
binding of these hormones to their receptors results in the
activation of phospholipase C to cleave phosphatidylinositol 4,5-
bis(phosphate) (PIP_2). This hormone-receptor regulated process
results in the formation of 1,2-diacylglycerol (DAG) and inositol

1,4,5-tris(phosphate) (IP$_3$), two compounds identified as "second messengers", which in turn regulate a wide variety of metabolic processes. Among the agents which induce PIP$_2$ hydrolysis are histamine, angiopressin, and a number of growth factors such as bombesin and platelet-derived growth factor. [The biochemistry of phosphatidylinositol metabolism has been recently reviewed (15), as has the relationship of PIP$_2$ hydrolysis to growth regulation (14, 16).]

The enzymic reactions of phosphatidylinositol (PI) formation and hydrolysis are shown in Figure 1. The formation of PI from cytidinediphosphate diglyceride (CDP-diglyceride) and myo-inositol is catalyzed by PI synthetase (reaction a. in Figure 1). A fraction of the PI in membranes is then further phosphorylated sequentially at the 4-position by PI kinase, then at the 5-position by PIP kinase to yield phosphatidylinositol 4,5-bis(phosphate) (PIP$_2$). While PIP$_2$ represents only a small percentage (i.e., <10%) of the total PI's in cells, it is the crucial substrate for phospholipase C, which yields DAG that remains associated with the membrane, and IP$_3$, which diffuses into the cytosol (reaction d.). Both of these products can serve as second messengers for modulating a number of intracellular reactions. These cyclitol phosphates are recycled into PI by a series of discrete enzyme-catalyzed reactions. The key step in this sequence is the reaction catalyzed by phospholipase C, as this reaction is activated by growth factors and hormones in cells possessing the appropriate receptors.

The central role of phospholipase C in such important processes as platelet aggregation, inflammation, hormone secretion, and growth regulation suggest that the process of PIP$_2$ formation and hydrolysis, as shown in Figure 1, would be a good target for drug design. For example, an inhibitor of phospholipase C activity may inhibit the growth of cancer cells which are proliferating due to excess release of growth factors or to an an excess of growth factor receptors. It is important to note, however, that the toxicity of such an inhibitor may also be great, as the role of this process in normal physiology is not clear at present. Nonetheless, if selectivity can be achieved, inhibitors of this process have great promise in control of cell proliferation.

Our initial efforts in the design and synthesis of inhibitors of the phospholipase C signaling system have been the synthesis of analogues of myo-inositol (1) with specific substitutions of fluorine for hydroxyl groups at key locations on the cyclohexane ring. The compounds, which are modified at positions 2, 4, and 5 (myo numbering), are shown in Figure 2. These compounds were selected for initial synthesis and evaluation as they retained greatest structural similarity to myo-inositol (1), but, in the cases of C-4 and C-5 substitution, lacked the sites required for further phosphorylation. Thus these compounds were considered good candidates for incorporation into cellular phospholipid, i.e., these should be substrates for PI synthetase (reaction a, Figure 1). Once these are incorporated, it was considered that they might inhibit either PI kinase (reaction b), PIP kinase (reaction c), or phospholipase C (reaction d). Alternatively, if these functioned as

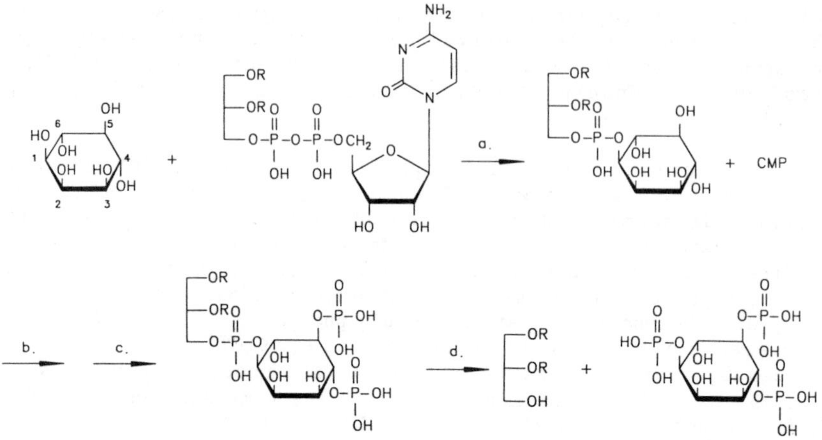

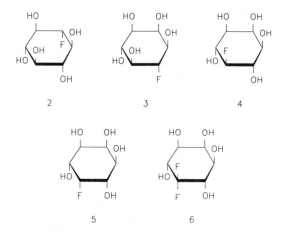

Figure 1.   Phosphoinositide Pathway.   Enzymes: a. phosphatidylinositol synthetase (PI synthetase); b. phosphatidylinositol
kinase (PI kinase); c. phosphatidylinositol-4-phosphate kinase
(PIP kinase); d. phospholipase C (R = palmitoyl or other long-
chain fatty acid chain).

Figure 2.   Target Deoxyfluorocyclitols: 1-Deoxy-1-fluoro-scyllo-
inositol (2); 4(6)-Deoxy-4(6)-fluoro-myo-inositol (3); 5-Deoxy-5-
fluoro-myo-inositol (4); 2-Deoxy-2-fluoro-neo-inositol (5); 5-
Deoxy-5,5-difluoro-myo-inositol (6).

substrates of phospholipase C, they might antagonize the action of the agonist because the product of phospholipase C action would not be IP$_3$, but would be the inactive analogue phosphates.

Results and Discussion

Chemical Syntheses.   Fluorination with diethylaminosulfur trifluoride (DAST).   The advent of the fluorinating reagent DAST (17) and its demonstrated effectiveness in the synthesis of deoxyfluoro carbohydrates (18) has greatly facilitated the direct fluorination of protected carbohydrate compounds.   The advantage of DAST over conventional fluorination reagents is the fact that it directly effects the fluoro-de-hydroxylation of R-OH compounds, without the intermediacy of an isolated sulfonate or other derivative bearing a leaving group.   (See eq. 1.)

$$R-OH + Et_2N-SF_3 \longrightarrow [R-OSF_2-NEt_2, \ F^-] \longrightarrow F-R + Et_2N-SF_2O^- \quad (1)$$

Generally, the fluorinated product is that of inversion (18), although examples of retention are known and have been attributed either to anchimeric assistance (19) or to steric crowding which prevents backside attack of F$^-$ on the intermediate (20).

1-Deoxy-1-fluoro-scyllo-inositol (2).   Preparation of this first target compound (see Figure 2) has been described by the Merck group (21).   Thus fluoro-de-hydroxylation of 1-O-benzoyl-3,4,5,6-tetra-O-benzyl-myo-inositol provided, after removal of the protecting groups, 1-deoxy-1-fluoro-scyllo-inositol (2).

4(6)-Deoxy-4(6)-fluoro-myo-inositol (3).   Syntheses of several other analogues have been documented in a recent paper that describes a number of deoxy- and deoxyhalogenocyclitols (22).   4(6)-Deoxy-4(6)-fluoro-myo-inositol (3, a racemic mixture of 4- and 6-fluoro derivatives) was synthesized (22) according to the scheme shown in Figure 3.   Fluorination of 3-O-benzyl-1,2,5,6-di-O-cyclohexylidene-myo-inositol (7) gave a ca. 4:1 ratio of myo- (8) and epi-isomers (9) as determined by ^{1}H NMR spectroscopy [J$_{3,4}$ = 3.7 and J$_{4,5}$ = 8.0 Hz for (8), and J$_{3,4}$ = 3.7 and J$_{4,5}$ = 4.4 Hz for (9).] That the major product was indeed that of retention was established upon deprotection (hydrogenolysis in acetic with palladium hydroxide on carbon) and examining the ^{1}H NMR spectrum of the product, 4(6)-deoxy-4(6)-fluoro-myo-inositol (3) and its penta-O-acetyl derivative 10.   For 3, J$_{3,4}$ = J$_{4,5}$ = 9.4 Hz, indicating a trans, diaxial arrangement of substituents in the H-3 - H-4 - H-5 portion of the molecule.   The resonance for H-4 of 3 appeared as a "doublet of pseudo triplets" with a wide spacing (J$_{H,F}$ = 53 Hz).   Attempted deprotection of 9 unfortunately resulted in product decomposition, possibly due to ready elimination of HF facilitated by the all-trans arrangement of H-3, F-4, and H-5.

5-Deoxy-5-fluoro-myo-inositol (4) and 2-deoxy-2-fluoro-neo-inositol (5).   Replacement of the hydroxy group with fluorine at the C-5 position of myo-inositol (1) is a very attractive goal, given the fact that such compounds should be nearly isosteric with 1 and would retain the internal symmetry inherent with the natural compound.   To

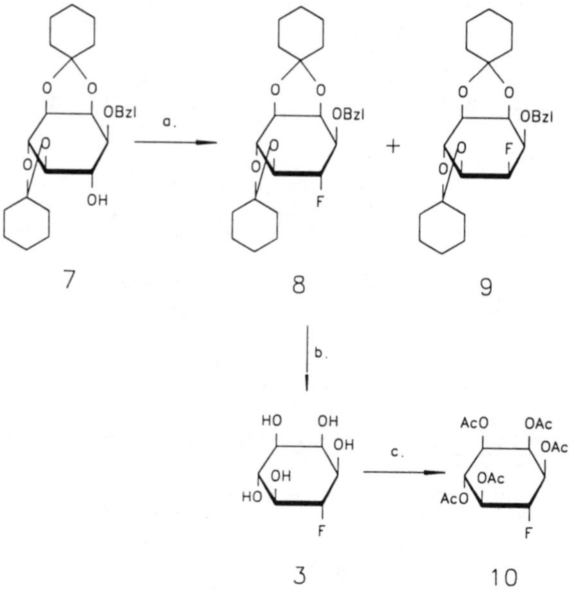

Figure 3. Synthesis of 4(6)-deoxy-4(6)-fluoro-myo-inositol (3).
Reagents: a. Diethylaminosulfur trifluoride (DAST); b. H$_2$ -
Pd(OH)$_2$/C, HOAc; c. Ac$_2$O - pyridine.

this end, 6-O-benzyl-1,2:3,4-di-O-cyclohexylidene-myo-inositol (11, Figure 4) was subjected to fluoro-de-hydroxylation with DAST to give the inverted product 12, along with the product of retention 13, in a ratio of 2.5:1. The two compounds were easily distinguished by their ^{1}H NMR spectra, with 12 showing for H-5 a wide doublet of doublets at δ5.10 ($J_{H,F}$ = 55.5, $J_{4,5}$ = ~0, and $J_{5,6}$ = 1.9 Hz). Unusually large vicinal H-F couplings were observed for H-4 (δ3.90 dd: $J_{H,F}$ = 28.2, $J_{3,4}$ = 3.9, and $J_{1,6}$ = 6.7 Hz). Thus an H-3 - H-4 trans geometry and an H-4 - H-5 - H-6 cis geometry are indicated for compound 12. Similarly, compound 13 was established to be of the myo-configuration with $J_{3,4}$ = 10.0, $J_{4,5}$ = 8.0, and $J_{5,6}$ = 7.7 Hz, respectively, showing the requisite all-trans geometry in the H-3 - H-6 portion of the molecule. Deprotection of compounds 12 and 13, as for the previous example, gave the free cyclitols 2-deoxy-2-fluoro-neo-inositol (5) and 5-deoxy-5-fluoro-myo-inositol (4), respectively, in excellent yields. Their ^{1}H NMR spectra (especially the spectrum of 5) were complicated by overlapping resonances; however, the H-4 - H-5 couplings were discernable, especially for their respective penta-O-acetyl derivatives 14 and 15 ($J_{4,5}$ = 2.0 and $J_{5,6}$ = 2.2 Hz for 14; $J_{4,5}$ = $J_{5,6}$ = 9.2 Hz for 15), indicating the cis geometry for the H-4 - H-5 - H-6 of 5 and 14 and the trans geometry for 4 and 15. Wide geminal proton-fluorine couplings (51 - 54 Hz) were present in all four compounds (for details see ref. 22).

Inasmuch as biochemical data (see discussion which follows and ref. 23) showed 5-deoxy-5-fluoro-myo-inositol (4) to be the most interesting compound among the 5-modified myo-inositols (22), and, given the fact that 4 is the minor isomer of the two produced in the sequence shown in Figure 4, a higher yielding process to 4 was sought. [The process shown in Figure 4 gives compound 4 in <1% overall yield from myo-inositol (1).]

Considering the available isomers of di-O-cyclohexylidene-myo-inositols, work has shown (24, 25) that 1,2:4,5-di-O-cyclohexylidene-myo-inositol (the precursor to 16, Figure 5) can be obtained in ca. two-fold higher yield than 1,2:3,4-di-O-cyclohexylidene-myo-inositol, the immediate precursor to 11. Thus the former intermediate was selected, and a route to 4 was developed from it (Figure 5). Benzylation of 1,2:4,5-di-O-cyclohexylidene-myo-inositol, using phase-transfer techniques (24), gave the 3,6-di-O-benzyl derivative 16 (22, 26), which was selectively deprotected at the C-4 - C-5 positions using ethylene glycol - p-toluenesulfonic acid (27) to give the diol 17 (28). Benzylation, again using phase-transfer techniques, produced a ca. 1:1 mixture of monobenzylated 18 and 19 which were chromatographically separated and crystallized in 75% yield. Compound 18 was then converted to its trifluoromethane-sulfonyl derivative, which without purification was reacted with cesium propionate (29) in N,N-dimethylformamide (DMF) to give the 5-O-propionyl-neo-analogue 20. Hydrolysis of the ester produced 1,3,4-tri-O-benzyl-5,6-O-cyclohexylidene-neo-inositol (21), a stable intermediate which has shown considerable utility in the synthesis of numerous 5-deoxy-5-modified inositols (22). Fluoro-de-hydroxylation of 21 with DAST, assisted by the addition of N, N-dimethylaminopyridine (DMAP) (30), gave the protected 5-deoxy-5-fluoro-myo-inositol (22) in 61% yield. Hydrogenolysis of 22 in

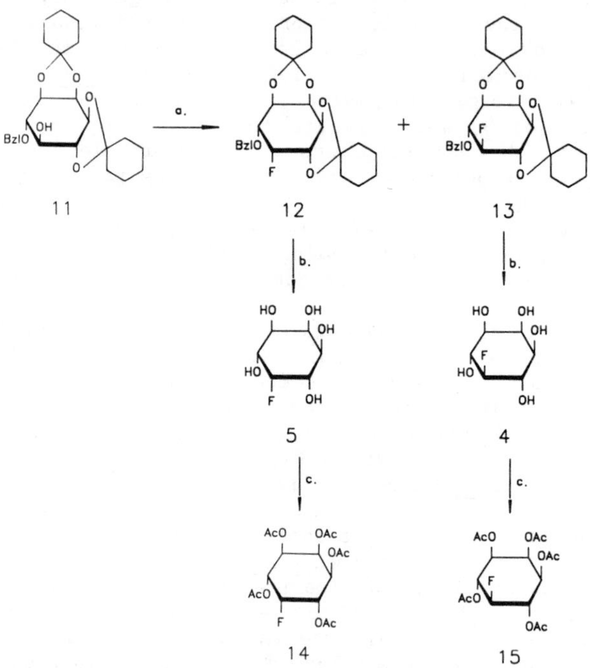

Figure 4. Synthesis of 5-deoxy-5-fluoro-<u>myo</u>-inositol (**4**) and 2-deoxy-2-fluoro-<u>neo</u>-inositol (**5**). Reagents: a. Diethylaminosulfur trifluoride (DAST); b. H_2 - $Pd(OH)_2$/C, HOAc; c. Ac_2O - pyridine.

acetic acid gave an 85% yield of the desired 5-deoxy-5-fluoro-myo-inositol (4) after crystallization. The product so obtained was identical in all respects with 4 produced by the alternative process (see Figure 4 and discussion in foregoing paragraphs). [Details of this improved synthesis of 5-deoxy-5-fluoro-myo-inositol (4) are to be reported. (Jiang, C.; Zayed, A.-H. A.; Baker, D. C., manuscript in preparation.)]

Radiolabeling of 5-deoxy-5-fluoro-myo-inositol (4). In order to provide a compound for in-depth biological evaluation, a radiolabeled derivative of 5-deoxy-5-fluoro-myo-inositol (4) was required. Using the method initially reported by Angyal and Odier for deuterium exchange on inositols (31), it was demonstrated that 4 could be cleanly exchanged with deuterium in deuterium oxide with Raney nickel as catalyst. By limiting reaction time (40 min) and temperature (60 - 65 °C), formation of isomeric byproducts was minimized. Examination of the recrystallized product so obtained by ^{1}H NMR spectroscopy revealed that 95% of the protium had been exchanged at the equatorial C-2 position, with lesser amounts (ca. 65%) of deuterium incorporation being observed at the C-1 and C-3 positions. Examination of the product by gas-liquid chromatography (GLC) showed >99% of pure, deuterium-exchanged 4. Using the conditions developed for deuteration, Moravic Biochemicals (Brey, CA) prepared a tritium-labeled product that was suitable for biochemical work. The tritium-labeled product was shown to be identical with unlabeled 4 and free of isomeric impurities by thin-layer chromatography (TLC) on cellulose plates in two systems (6:4:3 n-butanol - pyridine - water and 5:1 acetone - water) and on silica gel G in one system (2:1:1 n-butanol - acetic acid - water). The radiochemical purity of 4 indicated by these systems was >98%, and no detectable myo-inositol (1) was found. [Details of the exchange of protium with deuterium and tritium are to be reported. (Jiang, C.; Moyer, J. D.; Baker, D. C., manuscript in preparation.)]

5-Deoxy-5,5-difluoro-myo-inositol (6). Molecular modeling was used to assess the relative excluded volumes of various 5-substituted myo-inositols (23), and, judging from the results, it was deemed worthwhile to synthesize 5-deoxy-5,5-difluoro-myo-inositol (6). To this end, the versatile intermediate 18 was oxidized with chromium trioxide - dipyridine to give 1,4,6-tri-O-benzyl-2,3-O-cyclohexylidene-myo-5-inosose (23), which was subsequently fluorinated with DAST at 60 °C to give the gem-difluoro analogue 24 in 51% yield (Figure 6). Deprotection of 24 was effected with palladium hydroxide under 65 psi of hydrogen in acetic acid to give 5-deoxy-5,5-difluoro-myo-inositol (6) in 82% yield. ^{1}H NMR spectroscopy confirmed the meso compound's structure as 6: δ3.67 (2H, dd, $J_{3,4}$ = $J_{1,6}$ = 10.3 Hz, H-1, H-3), 3.99 (2H, ddd, $J_{4,F}$ (trans) = $J_{6,F}$ (trans) = 21.6 Hz; $J_{H4,F}$ (cis) = $J_{6,F}$ (cis) = 4.8 Hz, H-4, H-6), 4.10 (1H, ψt, $J_{1,2}$ = $J_{2,3}$ = 3.1 Hz, H-2). Anal. Calc'd for $C_6H_{10}F_2O_5$: C, 36.01; H, 5.04; F, 18.99. Found: C, 35.94; H, 5.08; F, 19.01.

Biological Results. Incorporation of these analogues of myo-inositol (1) (see Figure 2) into phospholipid would be expected to be a prerequisite for activity as an inhibitor of either the PI

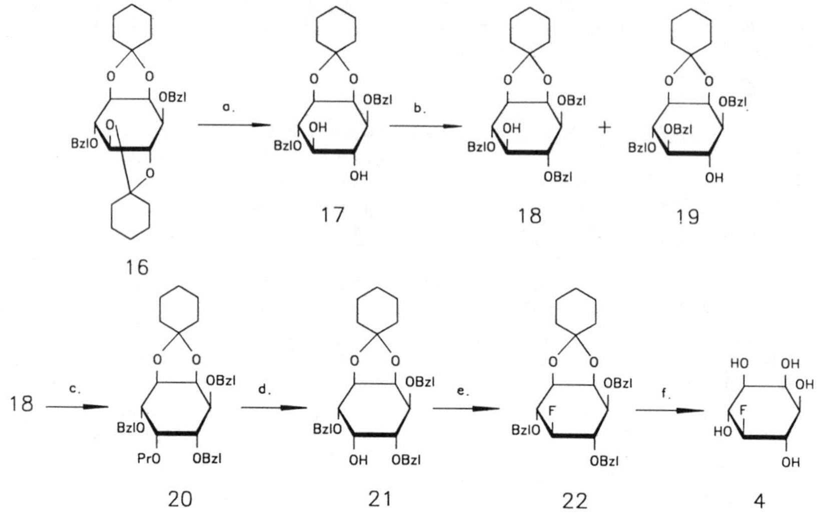

Figure 5. Improved synthesis of 5-deoxy-5-fluoro-myo-inositol (4). Reagents: a. p-TsOH, HOCH$_2$CH$_2$OH; b. PhCH$_2$Br - n-Bu$_4$NHSO$_4$/NaOH; c. (CF$_3$SO$_2$)$_2$O - Pyridine; CsO$_2$CCH$_2$CH$_3$ - DMF; d. NaOH - MeOH; e. Diethylaminosulfur trifluoride (DAST) - DMAP; f. H$_2$ - Pd(OH)$_2$/C, HOAc.

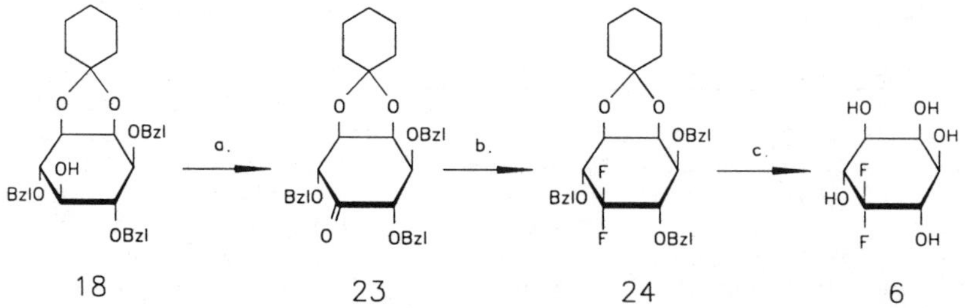

Figure 6. Synthesis of 5-deoxy-5,5-difluoro-myo-inositol (6). Reagents: a. CrO$_3$ - Pyridine - Ac$_2$O; b. Diethylaminosulfur trifluoride (DAST); c. H$_2$ - Pd(OH)$_2$/C, HOAc.

kinase or phospholipase C, as the substrates for both enzymes are phospholipids containing myo-inositol and not free myo-inositol itself. Previous studies of PI synthetase had suggested that the requirements for the inositol substrate were very stringent (32, 33). Our results (Table I) revealed that either replacement, or replacement with inversion, of the hydroxyl at the 2 or 4(6) position with fluorine led to loss of all detectable ability of the analogue to be incorporated into phospholipid as assayed by the stoichiometric formation of CMP from CDP-diglyceride. [It is noteworthy that, since 3 is a mixture of 4- and 6-isomers, interpretation of the results for 3 is not straightforward as one isomer could be an inhibitor and the other a substrate. Results of a separate experiment (23) using [³H]myo-inositol, however, indicated that the racemic mixture was not an inhibitor of PI synthetase.]

Table I. Fluorinated myo-inositol analogues (2 - 6) as substrates for PI synthetase from rat brain[a]

Analogue (no.)	Substrate Activity CMP Formation (% of myo-inositol)
myo-inositol (1)	100
1-deoxy-1-fluoro-scyllo-inositol (2)	<5
4(6)-deoxy-4(6)-fluoro-myo-inositol (3)	<5
5-deoxy-5-fluoro-myo-inositol (4)	26 ± 4
2-deoxy-2-fluoro-neo-inositol (5)	16 ± 2
5-deoxy-5,5-difluoro-myo-inositol (6)	<5

[a] Each analog was incubated with 5 mM CDP-diglyceride and solubilized rat brain microsomes as a source of PI synthetase as described (34). The amount of CMP formed from CDP-diglyceride was determined by separation by anion exchange chromatography and quantitated by the absorbance at 280 nm. Each analog was present at 5 mM. The extent of CMP formation as a percent of that generated with 5 mM myo-inositol (1) as substrate is reported in the table for 10-min incubations. The rate for myo-inositol was 3.8 nmol/10 min. Each value is the mean SD for three or more determinations, and the results are representative of those found in at least three independent experiments.

On the other hand, substitution of fluorine at the 5-position, either in the axial (compound 5) or equatorial (compound 4) position, produced compounds that could serve as substrates, although at a lower efficiency than the natural substrate myo-inositol (1). (The relative substrate activities as shown in Table I were observed at 5 mM substrate concentration and may be different at other concentrations.) Interestingly 5-deoxy-5,5-difluoro-myo-inositol (6) was not a substrate. These studies indicated that analogues 4 and 5 could be incorporated into cellular phospholipids if they could gain access to the cell interior, but the extent of incorporation would be sensitive to the concentration of myo-inositol (1) intracellularly as they would have to compete with this more efficient physiological substrate. However, even in the presence of 5 mM myo-inositol (a 200-fold excess) a small degree of incorporation of 4 into phospholipid by PI synthetase was observed (Figure 7).

The ability of PI synthetase to use 5-deoxy-5-fluoro-myo-inositol (4) as a substrate was confirmed by use of a radiolabeled compounds as shown in Figure 7. PI synthetase incorporated the analog into lipid in a time-dependent manner. The incorporation was absolutely dependent on the presence of CDP-diglyceride and was inhibited by the presence of myo-inositol (1) in the incubation mixture, as expected for PI synthetase. Chromatography of the reaction mixture revealed that a single radiolabeled product was formed with a mobility similar to, but distinct from, that of PI. Subsequent analysis has shown that the product is converted to a water-soluble form on mild alkaline hydrolysis and yields 5-deoxy-5-fluoro-myo-inositol (4) on treatment with phospholipase D, in agreement with the formation of phosphatidyl-5-deoxy-5-fluoro-myo-inositol as the product (data not shown). Determination of the absolute structure of these phospholipids awaits large-scale enzymatic synthesis, isolation of the product, and studies by mass spectrometry and NMR spectroscopy.

Although the results with PI synthetase in vitro were encouraging, it was important to establish whether or not the analogues could be incorporated into cellular lipids by intact cells. A potential difficulty is the entry of the analogue into the cells because the plasma membrane could serve as a barrier. Studies by Majerus and coworkers had previously indicated that 5-deoxy-myo-inositol was excluded from $HSDM_1C_1$ mouse fibrosarcoma cells (35). However, we found that $[^3H]$5-deoxy-5-fluoro-myo-inositol (4) entered L1210 leukemia cells at a rate similar to that of myo-inositol (compare in Figure 8), and achieved an intracellular concentration similar to that of myo-inositol (1). Furthermore, this analogue was incorporated into cellular lipid, although at a lower rate (20%) than the rate of incorporation of myo-inositol (1).

Although the data described above show that replacement of a portion of the myo-inositol (1) present in cellular phospholipid with analogues 4 and 5 can be achieved, many questions remain about the potential of these compounds. We are currently studying the extent to which we can reduce the availability of PIP_2 to cells by pretreating with the analogues. Further studies will also determine

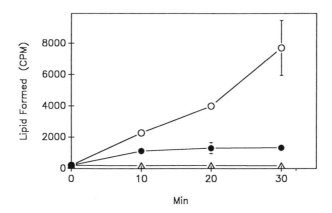

Figure 7. Incorporation of [³H]5-deoxy-5-fluoro-myo-inositol into lipid by PI synthetase of rat brain. [³H]5-deoxy-5-fluoro-myo-inositol (25 μM, 4 μCi/mL) was incubated with 5 mM CDP-diglyceride and solubilized rat brain microsomes at 37 °C as described in ref. 34. At the indicated times, 40-μL aliquots were removed, the reaction was terminated by the addition of trichloroacetic acid, and the lipid-soluble radioactivity was determined (o). Incubations without CDP-diglyceride (Δ) or in the presence of 5 mM myo-inositol (•) were also performed. The values shown are the mean +SEM for three independent incubations. This result is representative of three separate experiments.

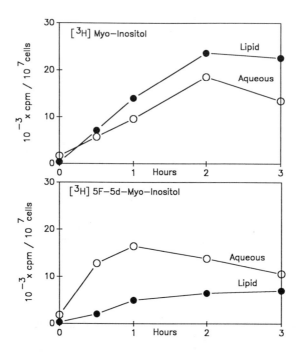

Figure 8. Incorporation of 5-deoxy-5-fluoro-myo-inositol (4) into intracellular pools and lipids of L1210 murine leukemia cells in culture. Exponentially growing L1210 cells were concentrated by centrifugation to 2 x 10^7 cells/mL in inositol-free Fisher's medium and incubated at 37 °C with 4 µCi/mL [³H]myo-inositol (upper panel) or [³H]5-deoxy-5-fluoro-myo-inositol (lower panel). The specific activity was 0.17 Ci/mmol for both compounds, and the concentrations were 25 µM. At the indicated times, samples of the cell suspension were removed, and the cells were collected by centrifugation through a layer of silicone oil and fractionated into lipid-soluble and water-soluble fractions. The values shown are the mean of duplicate incubations, and the result is representative of three independent experiments.

if these analogues can inhibit the formation of PIP and PIP_2 in cells or reduce the formation of second messengers when phospholipase C is activated.

Conclusions

The discovery of the role of PIP_2 hydrolysis in the action of a variety of hormones and growth factors has suggested a number of new targets for drug design. The fluorinated inositol compounds described herein are potentially of interest as inhibitors of key enzymes of phospholipid metabolism as they are capable of entering cells and becoming incorporated into phospholipid. Further work is needed to determine if these compounds can effectively inhibit the action of agents acting via the phosphoinositide pathway and whether there is a therapeutic usefulness for such inhibitors.

Acknowledgments

This work was supported, in part, by Contract No. N01-CM-27571 and Grant No. R01-CA-45796 from the National Cancer Institute of the National Institutes of Health.

Literature Cited

1.   Scherer, J. Liebigs Ann. Chem. 1850, 73, 322.
2.   Angyal, S. J.; McHugh, D. J. J. Chem. Soc. 1957, 3682.
3.   Posternak, T. The Cyclitols; Holden-Day: San Francisco, 1965.
4.   Fletcher, Jr., H. G. Adv. Carbohydr. Chem. 1948, 3, 45.
5.   Angyal, S. J.; Anderson, L. Adv. Carbohydr. Chem. 1959, 14, 135.
6.   Anderson, L. In The Carbohydrates; Pigman, W.; Horton, D. Eds.; Academic: New York, 1972, Vol. IA, p. 519.
7.   Anderson, R. J. J. Am. Chem. Soc. 1930, 52, 1607.
8.   Folch, J.; Woolley, D. W. J. Biol. Chem. 1942, 142, 963.
9.   Folch, J. Fed. Proc., Fed. Am. Soc. Exp. Biol. 1946, 5, 134.
10. Folch, J. J. Biol. Chem. 1949, 177, 497.
11. Folch, J. J. Biol. Chem. 1949, 177, 505.
12. Brockerhoff, H.; Ballou, C. E. J. Biol. Chem. 1961, 236, 1907.
13. Inositols and Phosphoinositides; Bleasdale, J. E.; Eichberg, J.; Hauser, G., Eds.; Humana: Clifton, NJ, 1985.
14. Berridge, M. J. Biochim. Biophys. Acta 1987, 907, 33.
15. Michell, R. H. Recept. Biochem. Methodol. 1986, 7, 1.
16. Berridge, M. J. Ann. Rev. Biochem. 1987, 56, 159.
17. Middleton, W. J. J. Org. Chem. 1975, 40, 574.
18. Card, P. J. J. Carbohydr. Chem. 1985, 4, 451.
19. Yang, S. S.; Beattie, T. R.; Shen, T. Y. Synth. Commun. 1986, 16, 131.
20. Castillion, S.; Dessinges, A.; Faghih, R.; Lukas, G.; Olesker, A.; Thang, T. T. J. Org. Chem. 1985, 50, 4913.
21. Yang, S. S.; Beattie, T. R.; Shen, T. Y. Tetrahedron Lett. 1982, 23, 5517.
22. Jiang, C.; Moyer, J. D.; Baker, D. C. J. Carbohydr. Chem. 1987, 6, 319.
23. Moyer, J. D.; Reizes, O.; Ahir, S.; Jiang, C.; Malinowski, N.; Baker, D. C., Mol. Pharmacol. 1988, in press.

24. Garegg, P. J.; Iversen, T.; Johansson, R.; Lindberg, B. Carbohydr. Res. 1984, 130, 322.
25. Jiang, C.; Baker, D. C. J. Carbohydr. Chem. 1986, 5, 615.
26. Angyal, S. J.; Russell, A. F. Aust. J. Chem. 1968, 21, 391.
27. Angyal, S. J.; Tate, M. E. J. Chem. Soc. 1961, 4122.
28. Hyertik, A. I.; Krylova, V. N.; Kozlova, S. P.; Klyashchitskii, B. A.; Shvets, V. I.; Evestigneeva, R. P.; Zhdavovich, E. S. Zh. Obshch. Khim. 1971, 41, 2747.
29. Kruizinga, W. H.; Strijtveen, B.; Kellogg, R. M. J. Org. Chem. 1981, 46, 4321.
30. Kováč, P.; Yeh, H. J. C.; Jung, G. L.; Glaudemans, C. P. J. J. Carbohydr. Chem. 1986, 5, 497.
31. Angyal, S. J.; Odier, L. Carbohydr. Res. 1983, 123, 13.
32. Benjamins, J. A.; Agranoff, B. W. J. Neurochem. 1969, 16, 513.
33. Agranoff, B. W. Fed. Proc., Fed. Am. Soc. Exp. Biol. 1986, 45, 2629.
34. Rao, R. H.; Strickland, K. J. Biochim. Biophys. Acta 1974, 348, 306.
35. Auchus, R. J.; Wilson, D. B.; Covey, D. F.; Majerus, P. W. Biochem. Biophys. Res. Commun. 1985, 130, 1139.

RECEIVED April 27, 1988

Chapter 5

Fluorinated Carbohydrates as Probes of Enzyme Specificity and Mechanism

Stephen G. Withers, Ian P. Street, and Michael D. Percival

Department of Chemistry, University of British Columbia,
Vancouver, British Columbia V6T 1Y6, Canada

The hydrogen bond strengths and polarities at each of
the sugar hydroxyls in the glycogen phosphorylase/
glucose complex have been determined through measurement of the affinities of a full series of deoxy and
deoxyfluoro analogues of glucose. Comparison of this
data with the recently refined X-ray crystal structure
of this complex reveals that the strongest hydrogen
bonds measured (≈ 3 kcal mol^{-1}) involve charged hydrogen
bond partners and that hydrogen bonds between neutral
partners contribute some 0.5 to 1.5 kcal mol^{-1}. The
electronegative fluorine substituent is also shown to
decrease rates of glycoside hydrolysis, presumably by
inductive destabilisation of oxocarbonium ion-like
transition states. Studies with fluorinated substrates
and glycogen phosphorylase have provided evidence for
an oxocarbonium ion mechanism and allowed estimation of
the strengths of hydrogen bonds involved in stabilising
the transition state. A novel mechanism-based inhibitor of β-glucosidases, 2,4-dinitrophenyl-2-deoxy-2-
fluoro-β-D-glucopyranoside, is also described. This
inhibitor works by rapidly glycosylating the enzyme but
only very slowly hydrolysing from the active site.

Deoxyfluoro- and deoxy-sugars are useful in studies both of binding
interactions between carbohydrates and proteins, and in mechanisms of
glycosyl transfer. This paper describes how we have used such
analogues to measure hydrogen bond strengths in a carbohydrate/
protein complex of known structure. It proceeds to review how such
substitutions affect the rates of glycosyl transfer in a
non-enzymatic model reaction and then applies this information to the
results obtained in our enzymatic system.
    There are a number of reasons why these analogues are useful.
Firstly the substitution of a sugar hydroxyl by a fluorine or by
hydrogen is sterically conservative since both these substituents are
smaller than the original hydroxyl. Table I provides the relevant

0097–6156/88/0374–0059$06.00/0

data and it is clear here that while fluorine is smaller than a hydroxyl it is considerably larger than a hydrogen when the bond length is taken into account; a point frequently overlooked in studies where fluorine is used as a replacement for hydrogen.

Table I. A Comparison of Size for Some Functional Groups
(Data from Reference 1)

GROUP	BOND LENGTH (Å)	VAN DER WAALS RADIUS (Å)	TOTAL (Å)
C-H	1.09	1.20	2.29
C-F	1.39	1.35	2.74
C-O(H)	1.43	1.40	2.83
C-OH	1.43	2.10	3.53

Secondly, the hydrogen bonding capabilities of these substituents vary considerably. The original hydroxyl, when optimally bound within a protein, can be involved in two hydrogen bonds as an acceptor (proton acceptor) and one hydrogen bond as a donor (see Reference 2 for some beautiful examples of such complexes). The hydrogen in a deoxy sugar cannot be involved in any significant hydrogen bonding. However, while the fluorine in a deoxyfluoro sugar cannot possibly donate a hydrogen bond, it can, arguably, act as a hydrogen bond acceptor (3). Thus the potential for hydrogen bonding is modified in an interesting way within such a series. The extent of involvement of fluorine attached to carbon, in hydrogen bonding is a matter of some debate. The high electronegativity of fluorine clearly favours bonding of this type, but since its lone pair electrons are held tightly to the fluorine nucleus it might be expected that the resultant hydrogen bonds would be somewhat weakened. Evidence for such hydrogen bonding in solution and in the gas phase does, however, exist. For example the relatively high boiling point of difluoromethane has been attributed (4) to intermolecular hydrogen bonding interactions involving fluorine. A similar explanation was provided for the observed dimerization of 2,2,2-trifluoroethanol in the gas phase (5). Better evidence for such hydrogen bonding interactions comes from X-ray crystallographic data. A recent review (6) of over 260 structures containing the C-F fragment revealed nine such interactions, the majority of which were C-F•••H-N hydrogen bonds. Two other more recent structures have shown the existence of C-F•••H-O hydrogen bonds in a fluorinated carboxylic acid (7) and in a difluorinated sugar (8). In the latter example (see Figure 1), both the fluorines were involved in weak, but significant, interactions as

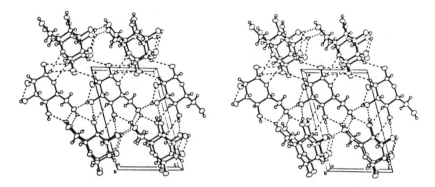

Figure 1. Stereoview of the packing of 2-deoxy-2-fluoro-β-D-mannopyranosyl fluoride. Broken lines represent hydrogen bonds and H•••(F/O) interactions with H•••F≤2.47Å and H•••O≤2.56Å. Letters a, b and c denote the unit cell axes defined elsewhere (Reprinted with permission from ref. 8. Copyright 1986 National Research Council of Canada.)

well as both the protons of the CHF fragments at C-1 and C-2. Thus
adequate evidence exists to suggest that the C-F fragment can indeed
act as a proton acceptor in a hydrogen bond. However, it is possible
that such hydrogen bonds involving fluorine may be more orienta-
tionally dependent than those on oxygen or nitrogen. These may then
only be observed as significant hydrogen bonds when the optimal
geometry is attained. This, however, would be the case for a
deoxyfluoro sugar replacing the native sugar in a protein binding
site, so such hydrogen bonds may be more significant than might
otherwise be expected.

It should, therefore, be possible to detect the presence of
hydrogen bonds to any individual hydroxyl by synthesising the
corresponding deoxy analogue and measuring its affinity for the
protein in question. The affinity difference should also provide
some measure of the contribution of that hydrogen bond to the overall
binding energy. It does not, however, give the full strength of that
hydrogen bond, as will be discussed below. Measurement of the
affinity of the corresponding deoxyfluoro sugar should provide
insight into the polarity of the hydrogen bond(s) in question. If
the original hydrogen bond involved the hydroxyl as a donor, then the
fluorine substituent cannot possibly participate, thus the
deoxyfluoro sugar should bind poorly. If, however, the hydroxyl acts
as an acceptor, then, since the fluorine can also act as an acceptor,
it may bind with similar affinity. Examples of both such cases will
be given later.

The full strength of the hydrogen bond is not measured under
such circumstances because it is also necessary to take into account
the competition of water for the hydrogen bonding sites (9). In
order to better understand the energetics of such interactions a full
hydrogen bond inventory must be performed (10-13). Thus, the
hydrogen bonding present at a single site in a ligand-protein
association in an aqueous medium can be expressed as in Equation 1
where the enzyme, E, has a hydrogen bond donor, H, which pairs with
the acceptor, A, of the ligand, L, in the complex.

$$E-H\cdots OH_2 + HOH\cdots A-L \Longleftrightarrow [E-H\cdots A-L] + HOH\cdots OH_2 \qquad (1)$$

These roles could, of course, be reversed.

Here two hydrogen bonds are seen on either side of the equation,
so both the numbers and types of hydrogen bonds are conserved in the
process, though geometry may well be different. The binding energy
expressed therefore results partially from enthalpic differences but
mainly from the increase in entropy associated with water release
into bulk water.

The removal of a hydrogen bonding group from the ligand L does
not lead to the loss of the full hydrogen bond energy as shown below
in Equation 2.

$$E-H\cdots OH_2 + HOH + L \Longleftrightarrow [E-H \, L] + HOH\cdots OH_2 \qquad (2)$$

Here, while there is no hydrogen bond in the enzyme-ligand complex,
there is no hydrogen bond from the ligand to water either, so only
one hydrogen bond appears on either side of the expression.
Experimentally, estimates of hydrogen bond strengths will be derived

from a comparison of the situations described in Equations 1 and 2.
Any energetic difference between such systems will not be equal to
the full hydrogen bond energy but to the differences in strengths of
hydrogen bonds formed with the protein and with water. These
differences could, however, be quite large when comparing a hydrogen
bond in an ordered, evolved, enzyme-ligand complex with that formed
between a relatively mobile water molecule and a protein residue.

Other Studies on Fluorosugar/Enzyme Interactions.

The glycosyl fluorides (fluorine at the anomeric centre) have been
investigated fairly thoroughly as substrates for their respective
glycosidases. The glycosidases studied are very specific for the
anomeric configuration of the glycosyl fluoride, with few exceptions
(14,15) and catalyse rapid hydrolysis of the sugar substrates. Such
substrates are frequently used in the enzymic synthesis of oligosaccharides by taking advantage of their enhanced transferase
activity (16). Additionally glucosyl fluorides have been the
substrate of choice for the polarimetric determination of the
stereochemical course of glycosidase hydrolysis (17). This method
takes advantage of the fact that glycosyl fluorides are generally
very good substrates for glycosidases (high V_{max}) and do not contain
a chromophore. The reaction course is followed polarimetrically and,
after a reasonable change in rotation has been observed, base is
added to stop the reaction and to rapidly mutarotate the product
formed. From the change in rotation upon base addition the anomeric
identity of the initial product is readily determined. Certain
α-glucan phosphorylases will also accept glycosyl fluorides as
substrates, in the presence of added phosphate (18).
     Sugars substituted with fluorine at non-anomeric centres have
found less general application, but have been used in a number of
specificity studies. Thus some excellent studies of the
specificities of a number of hexopyranose-binding enzymes were
completed at an early stage. These included yeast hexokinase (19)
and yeast galactokinase (20) where a full series of deoxyfluoro sugar
analogues was tested in each case. Hexokinase has been used to
synthesise a series of deoxyfluoro-glucose-6-phosphates (19,21,22).
These were then used in a study of yeast glucose-6-phosphate
isomerase (21) and of the glucose-6-phosphate dehydrogenases from
yeast and from rat liver (23). Almost all the analogues acted as
substrates, but at substantially reduced rates. Various other
studies have appeared since on enzymes such as galactose oxidase
(24), sorbitol dehydrogenase (25), UDP-glucose pyrophosphorylase
(26), gluconate dehydrogenase and gluconokinase (27), pyranose-2-
oxidase (28) and several other enzymes reviewed elsewhere (29). The
binding of fluorinated sugars to binding proteins such as lectins,
transport proteins and immunoglobulins has been studied in some
detail and used in formulating hypotheses regarding specific
interactions between the sugar and its protein binding site. This
material is covered by others in this book and so will not be
reviewed further here.
     Despite the number of studies performed on the binding of
fluorinated sugars to various proteins, there has never previously
been a systematic study of the binding of a full series of deoxy- and

deoxyfluoro-sugar analogues to a carbohydrate/protein complex whose detailed 3 dimensional structure has been determined by X-ray crystallography. Such an analysis is necessary to test the general validity of this approach, to evaluate hydrogen bond strengths and to relate these strengths to hydrogen bond types. The first part of this paper is concerned with such a study on the enzyme glycogen phosphorylase and its complex with glucose.

Hydrogen Bonding in the Glycogen Phosphorylase/Glucose Complex. A large number of deoxy and deoxyfluoro analogues of glucose were synthesised and these were tested (30) as inhibitors of rabbit muscle glycogen phosphorylase b, an enzyme known to be inhibited by glucose and whose 3-dimensional structure has recently been determined in the presence of D-glucose (31,32). The inhibition constants determined in this way represent true dissociation constants and are shown in Table II. Also listed is the composition of the pyranose anomers present as a percentage of the α-anomer. It is interesting to note that, with very few exceptions, and providing the anomeric centre is free to anomerize, the presence of substitution in the ring has very little effect on the anomeric ratios.

A detailed analysis of this data is presented elsewhere (30) but it is interesting to note the following points. Firstly the α-anomer of D-glucose is preferentially bound over the β-anomer (Ki $\approx$1 mM vs. $\approx$3 mM respectively) as determined by kinetic measurements performed (rapidly) on freshly dissolved samples of authentic α-D-glucose and β-D-glucose. This is reflected in the Ki values of α- and β-D-glucosyl fluoride and is consistent with the X-ray crystallographic observations (32). The 1-deoxy derivative (1,5-anhydro-D-glucitol) binds an order of magnitude more weakly than glucose, suggesting the presence of a hydrogen bond to the axial hydroxyl of glucose. Further, since α-D-glucosyl fluoride binds with approximately the same affinity as α-D-glucose, this suggests the presence of a hydrogen bond ($\approx$1.5 kcal mol^{-1}) in which the sugar hydroxyl acts as the acceptor. A similar situation obtains at the 2-position where the deoxy sugar binds $\approx$1.5 kcal mol^{-1} more weakly than D-glucose, but the deoxyfluoro sugar binds with the same affinity.

One major difference between the 1- and 2-positions is the response to inversion of configuration at each centre. Inversion at the 1-position ($\alpha \rightarrow \beta$) in the fluoro sugars results in loss of only $\approx$1 kcal mol^{-1} whereas inversion at the 2-position, best estimated in the difluorinated sugar series by comparing 2-deoxy-2-fluoro-α-D-glucosyl fluoride with 2-deoxy-2-fluoro-α-D-mannosyl fluoride, results in loss of 3.6 kcal mol^{-1}. Part of this decrease in binding energy at the 2-position (and probably all of it at the 1-position) is due to the loss of the specific hydrogen bond (1.5 kcal mol^{-1}) measured previously. This leaves 2.1 kcal mol^{-1} as the energetic cost of replacing the axial hydrogen with the bulkier fluorine. Thus an increase in size of approximately 0.5Å can lead to a severe binding energy decrease, suggesting a very specific complementary interaction at that site in the protein. Indeed, inspection of the recently-refined structure of the glycogen phosphorylase/glucose complex reveals a perfect van der Waals interaction between the hydrogen at C-2 and the carbonyl oxygen of the backbone amide of

Table II. Inhibition Constants for Glucose Analogues with Glycogen
Phosphorylase b + AMP*

No.	Name	Ki(mM)	Anomeric (%α) Composition
1	D-GLUCOSE	2.0	36
2	1-deoxy-D-glucose	10.7	N.A.
3	α-D-glucopyranosyl fluoride	0.6	100
4	β-D-glucopyranosyl fluoride	3.8	0
5	β-D-glucosylamine	10	0
6	2-deoxy-D-glucose	27	47
7	2-deoxy-2-fluoro-D-glucose	1.9	45
8	2-deoxy-2-fluoro-α-D-glucosyl fluoride	0.2	100
9	2-deoxy-2-fluoro-β-D-glucosyl fluoride	1.6	0
10	2-deoxy-2-fluoro-α-D-mannosyl fluoride	75	100
11	2-deoxy-2-fluoro-β-D-mannosyl fluoride	>>100	0
12	D-mannose	>>100	67
13	α-D-mannosyl fluoride	≈225	100
14	2-deoxy-2-fluoro-D-mannose	≈90	68
15	1,2-dideoxy-D-glucose	≈600	N.A.
16	3-deoxy-3-fluoro D-glucose	≈200	45
17	4-deoxy-4-fluoro D-glucose	25	41
18	6-deoxy-6-fluoro D-glucose	≈90	44
19	3-deoxy-D-glucose	>>100	25
20	4-deoxy-D-glucose	>>100	34
21	6-deoxy-D-glucose	>>100	45

*Ki values were determined by measurement of rates of phosphate
release from glucose-1-phosphate at five different substrate
concentrations around the Km value at each of five different
inhibitor concentrations. A Hill plot was used to extract apparent
Km values and these were replotted to give Ki values.

histidine 377. Any substituent larger than a hydrogen at this
position would result in a severe steric clash, which can only be
relieved by a protein conformational change involving movement of the
main chain residues.

The interactions with the 3-, 4- and 6-hydroxyls involve more
and stronger hydrogen bonds as evidenced by the fact that none of the
corresponding deoxy sugars binds at all. The corresponding deoxyfluoro sugars also bind much more poorly, but not as poorly as the
deoxy sugars showing that some of the hydrogen bonds are being
accomodated and further suggesting the presence of multiple hydrogen
bonds. On the basis of this data we have been able to predict the
following order of <u>observed</u> hydrogen bond strengths and the role
(donor (D) or acceptor (A)) of the sugar hydroxyl at each position.

$$3(D) \approx 6(D \text{ and } A) > 4(D \text{ and } A) > 2(A) \approx 1(A)$$

<u>Comparison with X-ray Crystallographic Data.</u> A list of the
residues involved in interactions with the glucose hydroxyls in the
phosphorylase/α-glucose complex is shown in Table III. It is
gratifying to note that all of the hydrogen bond polarities observed
by crystallography are consistent with those predicted by kinetics.
Further, it is of interest to note that the strongest hydrogen bonds
<u>measured</u> (3.2 and 2.6 kcal mol^{-1} respectively at OH-3 and OH-6),
involve amino acid side chains which are charged, or potentially
charged. The residue interacting with OH-3, Glu 672, is certainly
charged since it also interacts strongly with Lys 574 but the
histidine charge state is less certain. The hydrogen bonds involving
charged residues appear to be strong ($\approx$3 kcal mol^{-1}) while those
involving only neutral residues appear to be weaker ($\approx$0.5$\rightarrow$1.5 kcal
mol^{-1}). These are particularly interesting numbers since essentially
identical values have been measured (13) for another enzyme/substrate
complex, tyrosyl tRNA-synthetase plus substrate, by a complementary
method involving site-directed mutagenesis.

It is of further interest to note that the sugar binding site of
the L-arabinose binding protein (2) which binds its sugar four orders
of magnitude more tightly (Ki $\approx$ 10^{-7} M) than does phosphorylase, contains a large number of charged residues. Indeed the hydrogen bonds
measured in that system are considerably shorter and more numerous
than observed in phosphorylase. This protein, therefore, has evolved
a tight binding site of high specificity by incorporating a large
number of charged residues. Phosphorylase, however, has evolved a
binding site of high specificity, but of relatively low affinity, by
both incorporating steric constraints to prohibit the binding of
unwanted epimers and by constructing a network of weak hydrogen
bonds, using predominantly neutral hydrogen bonding amino acid
partners.

<u>Mechanistic Studies</u>

The mechanisms of glycosyl transfer catalysed by glycosidases and
α-glucan phosphorylases are thought to involve an intermediate
glycosyl oxocarbonium ion species, or at least a transition state
with significant oxocarbonium ion character as shown in Scheme 1.
Substitution of hydroxyl groups by the more electronegative fluorine

Table III.
HYDROGEN BONDING INTERACTIONS IN THE
GLUCOSE/PHOSPHORYLASE COMPLEX

SUGAR HYDROXYL	PROTEIN RESIDUE, ATOM INVOLVED, AND ITS ROLE AS DONOR (D) OR ACCEPTOR (A)
OH-1	Leu 136 N (D)
OH-2	Asn 284 ND2 (D)
	Tyr 572 OH
OH-3	Glu 671 OE2 (A)
	Ser 673 N (D)
OH-4	Asn 284 OD1 (A)
	Gly 674 N (D)
OH-6	His 376 ND1
	Asn 483 OD1 (A)

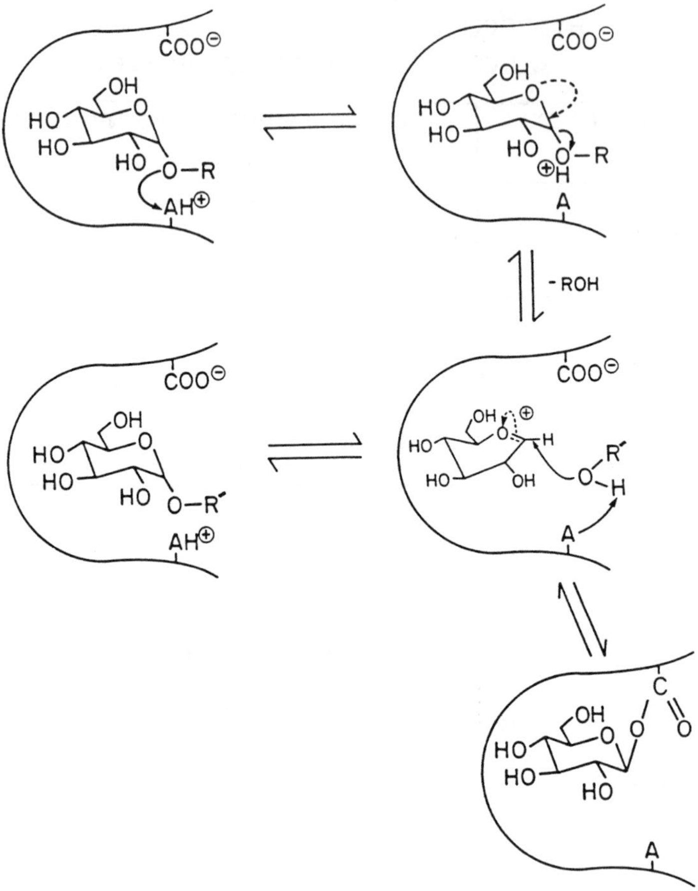

Scheme 1. General mechanism of α-glucosyl transferases. R may be one of a variety of aglycones. R'OH may represent water or the non-reducing terminus of an oligosaccharide.

atom, especially directly adjacent to the anomeric centre, should result in inductive destabilisation of such cationic species or states. This should result in an overall decrease in the turnover rate. The converse should be true for deoxy sugars, thus these should turnover more rapidly based on this criterion.

As a test for this we have studied a model reaction, the acid-catalysed hydrolysis of a series of deoxyfluoro-D-glucopyranosyl phosphates. Acid-catalysed hydrolysis of the parent sugar phosphate was demonstrated previously to proceed via an oxocarbonium ion intermediate by Bunton et al. (33,34) who also determined the mechanism of bond cleavage at a variety of pH values. More recent work (35) addressed the effects of structural changes in the sugar on the rate of acid-catalysed hydrolysis of its 1-phosphate. The results were seen to be consistent with those obtained for the acid-catalysed hydrolysis of equivalent alkyl and aryl glucopyranosides (36-38).

We have measured the first order rate constants for the acid-catalysed (1M HClO$_4$) hydrolysis of the series of deoxyfluoro-D-gluco-pyranosyl phosphates and these are given in Table IV.

Table IV. Acid Catalysed Hydrolysis Data

Compound	Hydrolysis Temperature (°C)	Rate Constant $k_o \times 10^5$ sec^{-1}
α-D-glucopyranosyl phosphate	25	4.10
6-deoxy-6-fluoro-α-	25	1.12
4-deoxy-4-fluoro-α-	25	0.270
3-deoxy-3-fluoro-α-	25	0.480
2-deoxy-2-fluoro-α-	25	0.068
2-deoxy-2-fluoro-β-	25	0.175

Clearly fluorine substitution has, in each case, lowered the rate relative to that of the parent compound, with the greatest rate depression (60-fold) being for the 2-substituted analogue. A more detailed discussion of these results is presented elsewhere (39) but it is interesting to note that the order of rates of hydrolysis is 6-fluoro > 3-fluoro > 4-fluoro > 2-fluoro, which is the inverse of the order observed for the acid-catalysed hydrolysis of series of alkyl (40) and aryl (41) deoxy β-D-glucopyranosides (i.e. 2-deoxy > 4-deoxy > 3-deoxy > 6-deoxy). This inverse relationship suggests a common, probably electronic, origin and we provide two possible

rationales as follows. Clearly inductive effects will be important
at the 2-position, but these would be expected to be attenuated
rapidly with distance from the anomeric centre. They might, however,
be sufficient to at least partially explain the observed order of
rate constants if one assumes that the majority of the positive
charge in the oxocarbonium ion resides on the ring oxygen. In that
case the 4-substituent is closer to the charge than is the 3-position
so its effect should be greater. However, the 6-position is also
just as close, yet the 6-fluoro derivative hydrolyses more rapidly
than the 3-fluoro compound. Another possible explanation relates to
the relative orientation of dipoles associated with C-OH and C-F
bonds in the ground state and in the half chair transition state,
since increased alignment of dipoles at the transition state would be
expected to result in rate decreases. The importance of such dipolar
interactions has been amply illustrated by the anomeric effect. As
detailed elsewhere (39), there is an overall decrease in dipolar
alignment for the 3-fluoro sugar in going to the transition state
which should increase its rate relatively, whereas substitution at
the 2- and 4-positions results, respectively, in an increase in
alignment and in no net change. The result of this would be to
decrease the rate of the 2-fluoro relatively and to leave the
4-fluoro slower than the 3-fluoro. This could be the cause of the
order inversion and the converse would clearly follow for the
deoxyglucosides. In reality both effects probably contribute.

The activation entropy and enthalpy were determined for the
2-fluoro analogue ($\Delta H^{\neq}$ = 113.5 k J mol^{-1}; $\Delta S_{25}^{\neq}$ = 4.0 eu) and compared
with those ($\Delta H^{\neq}$ = 116.6 k J mol^{-1}; $\Delta S_{25}^{\neq}$ = 14.9 eu) for the parent
sugar phosphate (33). Surprisingly, the major difference is in the
activation entropy which suggests a more S_N2-like transition state
involving considerable preassociation of the water to the glycosidic
carbon atom. This is quite consistent with current suggestions
(38,42) that all solvolyses at sugar anomeric carbons proceed through
a pre-association mechanism and also with the recent observations
(43) of inductive enhancement of pre-associative participation in
other displacement reactions. Clearly, therefore, electronic effects
can be very important, but the magnitude of the electronic effects
observed in any case may not be predictable since the transition
state structure can vary considerably. This will be particularly
true, and hard to evaluate, at an enzyme active site.

Enzyme Studies: Glycogen Phosphorylase.

We have now studied fluorinated sugars as substrates of a number of
glycosyl transferases; our most complete study to date being with
rabbit muscle glycogen phosphorylase. This enzyme, which catalyses
the reversible phosphorolysis of glycogen, producing glucose-1-
phosphate is thought to operate via the elementary mechanism shown in
Scheme 1 (R = phosphate, R'OH = glycogen). As can be seen, binding
of glucose-1-phosphate is followed by the acid-catalysed cleavage of
the anomeric linkage liberating phosphate and producing a
carboxylate-stabilised glucosyl oxocarbonium ion intermediate, or
more likely a covalent glucosyl enzyme. Deglucosylation of the
enzyme, and consequent glucosyl transfer, will occur upon attack of
the 4-hydroxyl at the non-reducing terminus of glycogen. Thus both

the glucosylation and the deglucosylation of the enzyme are
considered to proceed via oxocarbonium ion-like transition states.
In light of this proposed mechanism it is of interest to
anticipate what would be the effects on turnover, of substituting
various sugar hydroxyls by hydrogen and by fluorine. Two major
effects come to mind, namely electronic effects and binding effects.

The previous study of the acid-catalysed hydrolysis of the
series of deoxyfluoro- and deoxy-α-D-glucose-1-phosphate analogues
has amply demonstrated the importance of electronic effects from such
substituents on reactions proceeding via cationic transition states.
As was seen in Scheme 1, this enzymic reaction is also thought to
proceed via oxocarbonium ion-like transition states. On the basis of
electronic effects alone, therefore, the deoxy substrates would be
expected to turn over more rapidly than the normal substrate and the
deoxyfluoro substrates more slowly.

Binding effects are somewhat more complex. As has been discussed many times previously (13,44,45), enzymes catalyse reactions
by specifically binding the reaction transition state structure,
thereby stabilising it and lowering the overall activation free
energy. Thus binding energy is used in a fairly direct way to effect
catalysis. Some very elegant studies involving protein mutagenesis
have been performed to measure the strengths of individual hydrogen
bonds involved in stabilising the reaction transition state for the
enzyme tyrosyl t-RNA synthetase (13,46). These studies suggested
that this enzyme takes advantage of the geometrical changes in the
substrate structure on approaching the transition state, to
selectively stabilize the transition state, thereby facilitating the
reaction. A similar situation may obtain with glycogen
phosphorylase, since the transition state oxocarbonium ion species
will have a half-chair conformation, distinctly different from the
ground-state chair conformation. Thus individual hydrogen bonds may
be very important in promoting such a transition. Any substitution
in the sugar ring which eliminates hydrogen bonds involved in
transition state binding will therefore result in lower turnover
rates. On this basis alone, therefore, the deoxy substrates should
be the slowest, since no hydrogen bonding is possible to the hydrogen
substituent. The deoxyfluoro substrates may be as poor as the deoxy,
but, on average, should be slightly better due to their capacity for
accepting hydrogen bonds.

These two factors, binding, and intrinsic electronic effects can
be expected, therefore, to combine and to affect rates of turnover.
Unfortunately, however, it is not a simple task to dissect these two
effects with any precision. Even though the intrinsic electronic
effects are known for a model reaction, the acid-catalysed hydrolysis
of the same compounds, these cannot be applied directly to the
enzymatic reaction since the absolute magnitude of such electronic
effects depends upon the precise transition state structure. It is
very unlikely that these transition state structures for the enzyme-
catalyzed and acid-catalyzed reactions will be identical.

Table V gives the Michaelis-Menten parameters, V_{max} and Km,
measured for turnover of these substrate analogues by rabbit muscle
phosphorylase b. V_{max}/Km values are used in this analysis since they
represent the second order rate for reaction of free enzyme and free
substrate which can be related to overall activation free energies.

Table V. Kinetic Parameters for Glycogen Phosphorylase b

COMPOUND	MUSCLE PHOSPHORYLASE b	
	$Vm/Km \times 10^{-4}$ $(L \cdot min^{-1}mg^{-1})$	$\Delta\Delta G^{\ddagger}$ $(kcal \cdot mol^{-1})$
G1P	187500	-
2-FLUORO G1P	1.08	7.3
3-FLUORO G1P	2.2	6.8
4-FLUORO G1P	37	5.1
6-FLUORO G1P	0.26	8.1
2-DEOXY G1P	n.d.	n.d.
3-DEOXY G1P	5.8	6.3
4-DEOXY G1P	400	3.7
6-DEOXY G1P	11.1	5.9

$\Delta\Delta G^{\ddagger}$ represents the difference in activation free energies of enzyme-catalysed reaction of glucose-1-phosphate and the respective analogue. This is calculated from Equation 3 where $(V_{max}/Km)_1$ is the value for glucose-1-phosphate and $(V_{max}/Km)_2$ is that for the analogue.

Clearly they are all very slow substrates which react at rates some 10^2 to 10^5 times slower than the normal substrate. Despite the aforementioned difficulties in dissecting the electronic and binding factors several important questions can be addressed as follows: (a) does enzymatic catalysis proceed via an oxocarbonium ion transition state? It was proposed earlier that, on the basis of binding factors only, the deoxy sugars should generally be worse substrates than the deoxyfluoro sugars. However, the converse is clearly seen to be true in comparing V_{max}/Km values. This can only be explained if the intrinsic electronic effects are important and the transition state has substantial oxonium ion character. These data therefore provide substantial support for the mechanism proposed. (b) How strong are the hydrogen bonds at the transition state? A minimum estimate of such hydrogen bond strengths can be obtained by considering V_{max}/Km values for the deoxy-sugar series. Since intrinsic electronic effects will tend to speed up their turnover, then any rate reduction observed must be due entirely to poorer binding at the transition state. The increases in activation free energy, $\Delta\Delta G^{\ddagger}$ can be readily calculated from Equation 3. These values are listed in Table V and are minimum estimates of the strengths of hydrogen bonds to the

$$\Delta\Delta G^{\ddagger} = RT \ln \frac{(V_{max}/Km)_2}{(V_{max}/Km)_1} \tag{3}$$

corresponding hydroxyl at the transition state. The values obtained are considerably larger than those measured in the study of glucose binding to the T-state enzyme. This is consistent with expectations regarding increased hydrogen bond strengths at the transition state. Further, it is clear that the hydrogen bonds at the 3- and 6-positions are the strongest, as was observed for glucose binding to T-state enzymes. This suggests a common glucose sub-site which remains intact during the T→R transition.

A Mechanism-Based Inhibitor for a β-Glucosidase. Glucosidase-catalysed hydrolyses are generally considered to proceed via a "lysozyme type" of mechanism similar to that discussed previously for glycogen phosphorylase and illustrated in Scheme 2 for a "retaining" glucosidase. Thus glucoside hydrolysis proceeds through some form of glucosyl-enzyme intermediate and via a transition state with substantial oxocarbonium ion character. On the basis of our previous studies we reasoned that substitution of the 2-hydroxyl by an electronegative fluorine should destabilise the transition states for glucosylation (k_1) and deglucosylation (k_2) of the enzyme, thus slowing down both these steps. However, further incorporation of a reactive leaving group as the aglycone into such deactivated substrates might increase the glucosylation rate sufficiently (without affecting the deglucosylation rate) to permit trapping of the 2-deoxy-2-fluoro-D-glucosyl enzyme intermediate. If the degluco-sylation rate is sufficiently slow this might permit isolation of an inactivated enzyme.
    Thus, 2,4-dinitrophenyl 2-deoxy-2-fluoro-β-D-glucopyranoside was synthesized by deprotection of its tri-0-acetate, which had been

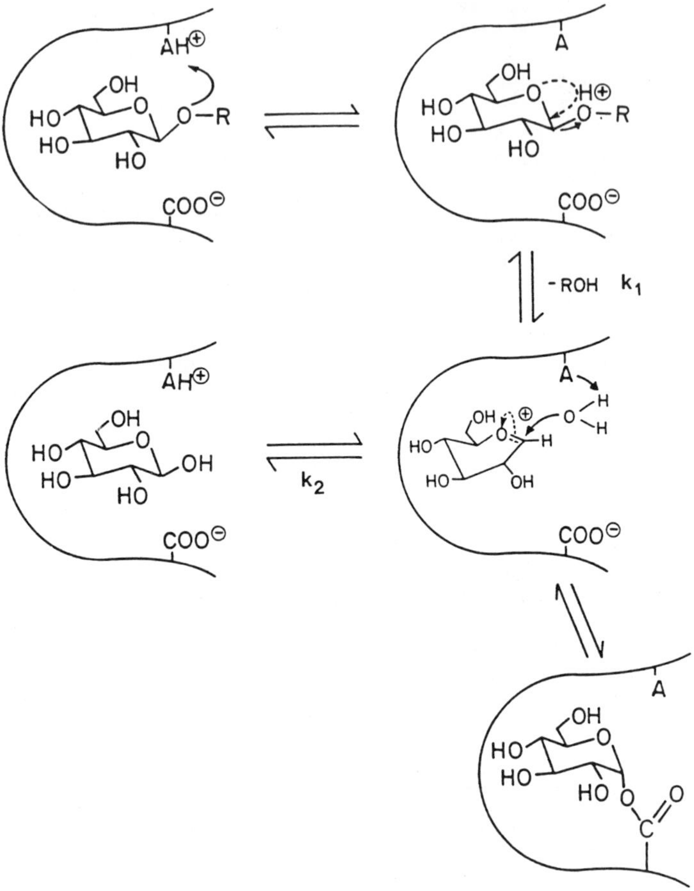

Scheme 2. General mechanism for β-glucosidases catalysing reaction with retention of configuration.

prepared by treatment of 2,3,6-tri-O-acetyl-2-deoxy-2-fluoro-D-glucopyranose with fluorodinitrobenzene, in the presence of base (1,4-diazabicyclo[2.2.2]octane) (47).   Incubation of Alcaligenes faecalis β-glucosidase (48) with this compound resulted in a rapid, time-dependent loss of enzyme activity. This followed pseudo-first-order kinetics as shown in Figure 2, permitting estimation of a dissocation constant (K_i) of 0.05 mM and an inactivation rate constant (k_i) of 25 minute^{-1}. The competitive inhibitor isopropyl-thio β-D-glucopyranoside provided protection against inactivation as shown in Figure 2, providing evidence that inactivation is due to reaction at the active site.

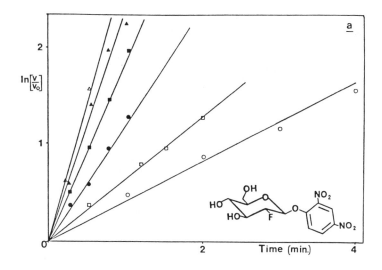

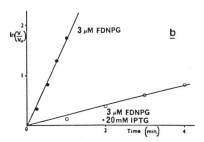

Figure 2.   Inactivation of <u>A. faecalis</u> β-glucosidase with 2,4-dinitrophenyl 2-deoxy-2-fluoro β-D-glucopyranoside.
a) Inactivation at the following inhibitor concentrations ($\bigcirc$ = 0.5 μM; $\square$ = 1.0 μM; $\bullet$ = 2.0μM; $\blacksquare$ = 3.0 μM; $\blacktriangle$ = 4.0 μM; $\triangle$ = 5.0 μM). b) Protection against inactivation given by isopropyl β-D-thioglucopyranoside. V_0 is the initial enzyme activity, V is the observed enzyme activity at the times indicated. Enzyme activity was measured by spectrophotometric assay of p-nitro-phenol release from p-nitrophenyl-β-D-glucopyranoside in 50 mM sodium phosphate buffer, pH 6.8.

This therefore represents a novel type of mechanism-based inhibitor of glycosidases which should be fairly generally applicable to this class of enzymes, provided that the deglycosylation rate for the analogue is sufficiently slow relative to the glycosylation rate. Experiments are currently planned to identify the active site nucleophile in this enzyme using such an inhibitor and to confirm its mode of action by purifying the inactive deoxyfluoroglucosyl enzyme and studying it by ^{19}F NMR. The general applicability of this approach is also being tested with a variety of glycosidases by use of the appropriate 2-deoxy-2-fluoro-glycoside in each case.

Conclusions

Suitable application of deoxy- and deoxyfluoro- analogues of enzymatic substrates has provided valuable insight into the mechanisms of enzyme-catalysed glucosyl transfer and into the role of hydrogen bonding in substrate recognition and catalysis. It has also permitted design of a novel class of mechanism-based enzyme inhibitors. Another appealing application of such compounds is their use in ^{19}F nmr studies of enzyme-substrate complexes. We have recently initiated such studies on the enzyme phosphoglucomutase.

Acknowledgments

This work was supported by grants from the Natural Sciences and Engineering Research Council of Canada and from the British Columbia Health Care Research Foundation.

LITERATURE CITED

1. Walsh, C. Adv. Enzymol. 1983, 55, 197.
2. Quicho, F.A.; Vyas, N.K. Nature 1984, 310, 381.
3. Barnett, J.E.G. In Ciba Fdn. Symp. Elsevier & Associated Scientific Press, Amsterdam, 1972; p95.
4. Sheppard, W.A.; Shantz, C.M. In Organic Fluorine Chemistry; W.A. Benjamin: New York, 1964; p 40.
5. Curtiss, L.A.; Frurip, D.J.; Blander, M. J. Am. Chem. Soc. 1978, 100, 79.
6. Murray-Rust, P.; Stallings, W.G.; Monti, C.T.; Preston, R.K.; Glusker, J.P. J. Am. Chem. Soc. 1983, 105, 3206.
7. Karipides, A.; Miller, C. J. Am. Chem Soc. 1984, 106, 1494.
8. Withers, S.G.; Street, I.P.; Rettig, S.J. Can. J. Chem. 1986, 64, 232.
9. Klotz, I.M.; Franzen, J.S. J. Am. Chem. Soc. 1962, 84, 3461.
10. Jencks, W.P. In Catalysis in Chemistry and Enzymology, McGraw Hill: New York, 1969.
11. Fersht, A.R. Trends Biochem. Sci. (pers. Ed.) 1984, 9, 145.
12. Hines, J. J. Am. Chem. Soc. 1972, 94, 5766.
13. Fersht, A.R.; Shi, J.P.; Knill-Jones, J.; Lowe, D.M.; Wilkinson, A.J.; Blow, D.M.; Brick, P.; Cortes, P.; Waye, M.M.Y.; Winter, G. Nature 1985, 314, 235.
14. Hehre, E.J.; Brewer, C.F.; Genghof, D.S. J. Biol. Chem. 1979, 254, 5942.
15. Kasumi, T.; Tsumuraya, Y.; Brewer, C.F.; Kersters-Hilderson, H.; Claeyssens, M.; Hehre, E.J. Biochemistry 1987, 26, 3010.

16. Treder, W.; Thiem, J.; Schlingmann, M. Tetrahedron Lett. 1986, 27, 5605.
17. Barnett, J.E.G. Biochem. J. 1971, 123, 607.
18. Palm, D.; Blumenauer, G.; Klein, H.W.; Blanc-Muesser, M. Biochem. Biophys. Res. Commun. 1983, 111, 530.
19. Bessell, E.M.; Foster, A.B.; Westwood, J.H. Biochem. J. 1972, 128, 199.
20. Thomas, P.; Bessell, E.M.; Westwood, J.H. Biochem J. 1974, 139, 661.
21. Bessell, E.M.; Thomas, P. Biochem. J. 1973, 131, 77.
22. Drueckhammer, D.G.; Wong, C.-H. J. Org. Chem. 1985, 50, 5913.
23. Bessell, E.M.; Thomas, P. Biochem. J. 1973, 131, 83.
24. Maradufu, A.; Perlin, A.S. Carbohydr. Res. 1974, 32, 93.
25. Taylor, N.F.; Romaschin, A.; Smith, D. In Biochemistry Involving Carbon-Fluorine Bonds, ACS Symposium Series 1976, 28, 99.
26. Wright, J.A.; Taylor, N.F.; Brunt, R.V.; Brownsey, R. J. Chem. Soc., Chem. Commun. 1972, 691.
27. Taylor, N.F.; Hill, L.; Eisenthal, R. Can. J. Biochem. 1975, 53, 57.
28. Squire, S.; Taylor, N.F. Proc. Can. Fed. Biol. Soc. Abstr. 1985, 28, 226.
29. Penglis, A. Adv. Carb. Chem. Biochem. 1981, 38, 195.
30. Street, I.P.; Armstrong, C.R.; Withers, S.G. Biochemistry 1986, 25, 6021.
31. Sprang, S.R.; Fletterick, R.J. J. Mol. Biol. 1979, 131, 523.
32. Sprang, S.R.; Goldsmith, E.J.; Fletterick, R.J.; Withers, S.G.; Madsen, N.B. Biochemistry 1982, 21, 5364.
33. Bunton, C.A.; Llewellyn, D.R.; Oldham, K.G.; Vernon, C.A. J. Chem. Soc. C 1958, 3574.
34. Bunton, C.A.; Humeres, E. J. Org. Chem. 1969, 34, 572.
35. O'Connor, J.V.; Barker, R. Carbohydr. Res. 1979, 73, 227.
36. Capon, B. Chem. Rev. 1969, 69, 407.
37. BeMiller, J.N. Adv. Carbohydr. Chem. 1967, 22, 25.
38. Sinnott, M.L. In The Chemistry of Enzyme Action, Elsevier: New York, 1984; p 389.
39. Withers, S.G.; MacLennan, D.J.; Street, I.P. Carbohydr. Res. 1986, 154, 127.
40. Overend, W.G.; Rees, C.W.; Sequeira, J.S. J. Chem. Soc. 1962, 3429.
41. Mega, T.; Matsushima, Y. J. Biochem. (Tokyo) 1983, 94, 1637.
42. Jencks, W.P. Chem. Soc. Rev. 1981, 10, 345.
43. Lambert, J.B.; Larson, E.G. J. Am. Chem. Soc. 1985, 107, 7546.
44. Pauling, L. Chem. Eng. News 1946, 24, 1375.
45. Fersht, A.R. In Enzyme Structure and Mechanism (2nd Edn.) W.H. Freeman 1985.
46. Fersht, A.R.; Leatherbarrow, R.J.; Wells, T.N.C. Trends Biochem. Sci. (Pers. Ed.) 1986, 9, 145.
47. Withers, S.G.; Street, I.P.; Bird, P.; Dolphin, D.H. J. Am. Chem. Soc. 1987, 109, 7530.
48. Day, A.G.; Withers, S.G. Biochem. Cell Biol. 1986, 64, 914.

RECEIVED March 14, 1988

Chapter 6

Deoxyfluoro Carbohydrates as Probes of Binding Sites of Monoclonal Antisaccharide Antibodies

Cornelis P. J. Glaudemans and Pavol Kováč

National Institutes of Health, Bethesda, MD 20892

The mode of binding of a β-(1→6)-D-galactopyranan
to a group of monoclonal antibodies is examined.
The combining area in these antibodies has four
subsites, each capable of binding to a single
galactosyl residue in a sequence of four in the
antigen. One subsite has the highest affinity for
its residue amongst the four, and that subsite
binds through H-bonding to the hydroxyl groups at
positions 2 and 3 of the galactosyl residue it
associates with. Thus, by using *galacto*
oligosaccharides bearing a 3-deoxyfluoro group at
defined positions, and thereby prohibiting the
binding of that (substituted) galactosyl residue to
the subsite with the highest affinity, the order of
the affinities of the four subsites could be
measured. Correlation of the binding data with the
amino acid sequences of the antibodies studied has
led to a proposal for the arrangement of the bound
antigen on the surface of the immunoglobulins. The
synthetic routes to a variety of the ligands used
is discussed in detail.

Immunoglobulins - or antibodies - are a class of proteins
secreted by plasma cells. The clonal selection theory, now
generally accepted, proposes that precommitted B-lymphocytes
(whose progeny is the plasma cell) have the specificity of the
immunoglobulin they produce, and which occurs on their cell-
surface in small amounts, encoded in their genome (1). An
immunogen, upon entering the body selects lymphocytes that carry
immunoglobulin of the appropriate specificity and then combines
with that immunoglobulin, thus stimulating the proliferation of
these cells. By a process not entirely understood, B-lymphocytes,
now stimulated by immunogen-contact, differentiate through a
lymphoblast into a plasma cell which produces large amounts of
immunoglobulin (2). The combination of immunogen with surface
immunoglobulin appears to be the driving force of this

differentiation, since B-lymphocytes can also be triggered to differentiate by cross linking their surface proteins with pokeweed mitogen (3). Since even a simple antigen usually has many structural determinants, it can combine with the surface immunoglobulins of a large number of different immunocompetent cells. Although each of these cells produces a single, unique immunoglobulin, the overall response would thus still yield a heterogeneous pool of immunoglobulins. It is true that some immune responses express themselves monoclonally (or nearly so), and thus produce a single molecular species of antibody (4,5), but the predominant source of monoclonal antibodies is through immunoglobulin-producing neoplasms, i.e. proliferative plasma cells or plasma cytomas (6-8). Originally, spontaneous, or randomly induced plasma cytomas were the major source of monoclonal antibodies. Thus, the monoclonal immunoglobulins (6,7) were screened for their specificities (9-12) and subsequent work led directly to an early insight into the process of the immune response, as well as to an understanding of the nature of antigen-antibody interaction. In 1965 Sach, Horibata, Lennox and Cohn began *in vitro* culturing of murine plasma cytomas (see reference 12 for a description of these events) and this led to the discovery by Köhler and Milstein (13) that plasma cytomas can be fused with normal plasma cells to yield a hybridoma producing monoclonal antibody of predetermined specificity. These hybridomas are pathologically proliferative, are transplantable, and form the basis for obtaining large amounts of immunoglobulins of desired specificity. As the number of monoclonal antibodies increased (12,14,15) they were used for a variety of studies including the elucidation of the genetics of the immune response. This article will bring up to date certain aspects of a previous review on this subject (16) as well as present a new method to elucidate the location of binding sites and sub-sites in monoclonal antibodies.

GENERAL FEATURES OF IMMUNOGLOBULINS

Several immunoglobulin fragments have been investigated by X-ray diffraction of their crystals (17-22). These studies have revealed that corresponding immunoglobulin domains generally have very similar structures. An excellent review has been published (22). In summary: Antibodies are made up of two identical heavy (H) chains of molecular weight *ca.* 50,000 Daltons, and two identical light (L) chains of molecular weight *ca.* 25,000 Daltons (23). These four chains form a number of globular domains, each domain containing approximately 100 amino acids. The N-terminal domains of of each H,L pair together harbor one combining site at the solvent exposed end of the molecule. Thus, each four chain unit H_2L_2 posesses two combining sites, and they are identical. The N-terminal domains of both the H and the L chain vary from immunoglobulin to immunoglobulin, while for a given class of immunoglobulins the remainder of the H and L chains are identical. The variability of the first N-terminal domain of both the H and L chain expresses itself as a unique specificity, and this variability resides particularly in certain areas within the domain called hypervariable regions (24). These are loops of

about half a dozen or so amino acid residues, and there are three
such regions in both the H and the L chain. When the
immunoglobulin α-carbon backbone is observed it is noted that
these hypervariable (hv) loops, although separated in sequence,
occur near one another in space, and can together make up the
combining site (24). Diversity of immunoglobulins arises by
several ways (25), mostly at the genetic level (26-28), and it
would be inappropriate to discuss this here. Suffice it to say
that enormous diversity can be generated, but it must be
remembered that variations in amino acid sequence do not always
lead to changes in binding specificity.

Cohn originally described a myeloma immunoglobulin A (9)
which precipitated with the species-specific cell wall-teichoic
acid occuring in *Streptococcus Pneumoniae*. The haptenic
determinant turned out to be phosphoryl choline and, since then,
innumerable myeloma and hybridoma monoclonal antibodies with
this specificity have been described (29-31). An anti-
phosphorylcholine IgA (Mc603) is one of the three immunoglobulins
whose structure has been solved by X-ray diffraction studies
(17,19,22,32,33). Thus, detailed knowledge of the three-
dimensional structure of its combining site, and the interaction
of the site with the ligand, has become the focal point of our
knowledge about the subject. In observing the combining site of
Mc603 it can be seen that the cavity is defined by the
surrounding surfaces formed by the hypervariable (hv) loops on
the face of the IgA. The first hv region of the L chain (hv_L-1)
is unusually long, and prevents hv_L-2 from reaching the cavity.
In addition, both hv_H-2 and hv_H-3 are longer than usual, and the
overall effect is the creation of a deep cavity. This is not a
general feature for immunoglobulins, and in the anti-galactan
monoclonal antibodies these hv regions are shorter, thereby
creating a shallower combining area (33).

ANTI-GALACTAN MONOCLONAL ANTIBODIES

One of the largest groups of monoclonal murine immunoglobulins
with anticarbohydrate specificity is the group of anti-galactans.
In addition to the myeloma immunoglobulins (14,16), a large
number of anti-galactan hybridoma immunoglobulins have been
elicited (34). One of the major areas that our laboratory has
worked on in the past years are these monoclonal immunoglobulins
with specificity for β(1→6)-D-galactopyranan (7,35-37).
Considerable progress has been made in the elucidation of details
of the interaction of that antigen with antibody, but these
details are far from complete. This is partly due to the fact
that - although X-ray diffraction studies of one of these
antibodies (J539 Fab') has been reported (33) - no crystals from
these antibodies have been obtained with the antigenic
determinant occupying the complementarity determining region
(38). We have shown that one of the members of this group, IgA
J539, binds along the length of the chain (intercatenarily) to
its linear β(1→6)-D-galactopyranan antigen (39), and the antibody
makes contact with four sequential galactosyl residues (40,41).
The areas of importance to binding in the *antigenic determinant*
have been mapped for two immunoglobulins in this group (J539 and

X24), and it has been shown that the antibody's highest binding subsite interacts with the C1-C2-C3 face of the galactosyl residue it binds (40-42). This laboratory proposed that the β(1→6)-D-linked galactobiose ligand, which binds to the antibody, is in a conformation having its ring oxygens on opposite sides of the disaccharide. In that conformation the galactobiose would bind with only one side to the antibody (41, see Fig. 1). In addition, derivatives of methyl β-D-galactopyranoside carrying

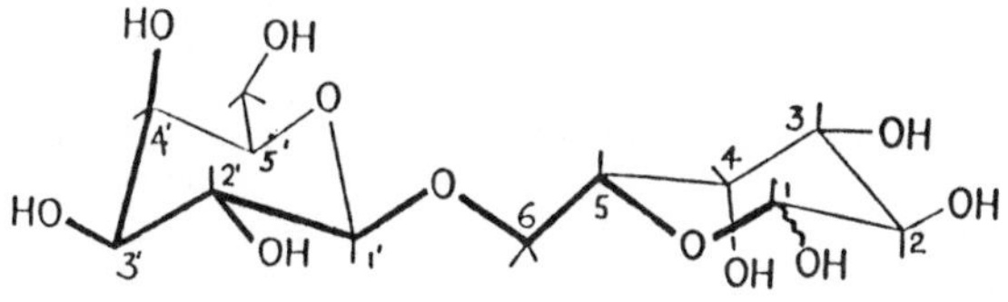

Fig. 1. The postulated conformation of 6-*O*-β-D-galactopyranosyl-D-galactose . [The heavy bonds indicate the area of strongest binding to the immunoglobulin A J539 (Fab').]

bulky substituents on C6 bound as did the unsubstituted sugar, indicating that the highest binding subsite was not spacially restricted, and probably was on the surface of the protein (42). The amino acid sequences of the variable part of both the H and the L chain of immunoglobulins of this group have been reported (28,34,43). In addition, it has now been shown that this entire group of antibodies is derived by somatic mutation operating on two genes v_HGal 39.1 and v_HGal 55.1 (44). Data obtained from affinity labeling may not always be useful, since the area around the site of protein-attachment would be equal in radius to the length of the ligand, it would quickly exceed the known area-size for the combining site of antibodies. We are nevertheless pursuing that approach (45-48), and the use of extremely reactive, indiscriminate (photo)affinity labels, such as diazirino glycosides of β-galactose is showing great promise (48). Most of our *present* insight results from our work on chemically altered ligand probes (40-42) culminating in the use of galactosyl (oligo)saccharides bearing fluorine in the place of hydroxyl groups at defined positions (49) to probe the possibility of hydrogen-bonding (50). This has led to the mapping of subsites in the combining area of antigalactan IgA J539 (35-37). Thus, if hydrogen-bonding indeed takes place, and if the *protein* were the hydrogen donor in bonding with any oxygen atoms in the sugar molecule, replacement of the hydroxyl groups involved by fluorine could increase the affinity for the hydrogen-bonding due to the higher electronegativity of the fluorine. If, on the other hand, hydrogen bonding should occur through hydrogen donation by a *sugar* hydroxyl group to the protein, synthetic carbohydrate-ligands bearing deoxyfluoro groups at the required position would probably show greatly diminished binding (or none at all). Should hydrogen bonding not be mediated by any of the hydroxyl groups substituted by fluorine in the D-galactoside, the affinities would probably not be greatly affected. It had been mentioned above that we had shown that the antibody combining area can accommodate four sequential galactopyranosyl residues, and that the antibody binds to interchain β(1→6)-linked tetrasaccharide segments of galactopyranans (39). It is to be expected that these four antibody subsites each have their own, differing affinity for "their" galactosyl residue, since the protein in general - including the combining area - has an anisotropic nature. Examination of the data presented in Table I permits an assignment of the relative strength of interaction of each antibody subsite with its galactosyl residue, and also permits a conclusion about the direction of the polysaccharide chain when it is bound to the antibody combining area. Considering only the spacial exclusion for each atom, we proposed a conformation for β(1→6)-D-galactooligosaccharides (or polysaccharides) having the ring oxygen of each residue in alternate fashion on opposite sides of the polysaccharide chain (41). Since then we have made energy-minimization (HSEA, 51) calculations (we are grateful to Dr. Klaus Bock for assisting us) for the tetrasaccharide O-β-D-galactopyranosyl-(1→6)-O-β-D-galactopyranosyl-(1→6)-O-β-D-galactopyranosyl-(1→6)-β-D-galactopyranose (see Fig. 2). This hypothetical conformation, which may or may not be the one the

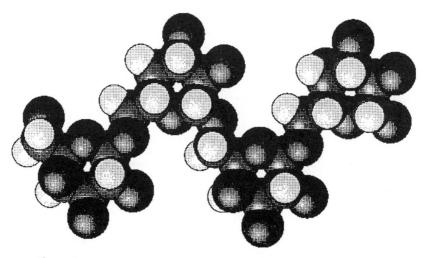

Figure 2.

Intersaccharidic bond angles for β-(1→6)-linked β-D-galactopyranotetraose as calculated by the HSEA method (51).

	ϕ	ψ	ω
Link 1	- 64.2°	- 171.7°	65.4°
Link 2	- 62.7°	- 164.2°	65.8°
Link 3	- 66.5°	179.5°	62.4°

oligosaccharide assumes when *actually* bound to the antibody, is used in this chapter to illustrate the binding mode of saccharide ligands to the monoclonal antibodies in our following discussion. A tetrasaccharide segment in this conformation has a linear dimension of *ca.* 17 Å. The subsite with the highest affinity for a galactosyl residue is likely to be near a solvent exposed tryptophanyl residue, since even the simplest ligand - methyl β-D-galactopyranoside - (5 in Table I) shows ligand-induced antibody tryptophanyl fluorescence change (41; for a detailed description of using ligand-induced changes of the antibody tryptophanyl fluorescence to measure affinity constants, see ref. 52). On the basis of an examination of the coordinates of IgA J539 Fab' obtained by X-ray diffraction studies at 2.7 Å resolution (33), it can be seen that the two tryptophanyl residues in the complementarity determining regions (CDRs, see ref. 38) of IgA J539, namely tryptophan (TRP) 33H and TRP 91L (28,38,53) appear solvent exposed (TRP 91L is partly solvent exposed) and are at the H/L interface in the center of the immunoglobulin combining area. These two TRP residues are separated by *ca.* 9-10 Å. The only other tryptophanyl residues near the *general* combining area, TRP 36H and TRP 35L, are not in the CDR and are buried where they would not be expected to be perturbable by ligands bound on the protein surface. The first antibody subsite to attract all or part of the ligand appears to be near TRP 33H, since a heterologous H/L-chain recombinant immunoglobulin we prepared (54), derived from the two anti-galactan IgA's S10 and J539, showed fluorescence characteristics upon binding methyl β-D-galactopyranoside similar to those of the H-chain donor-protein. Both immunoglobulins S10 and J539 have the invariant TRP 33H residue (53, J. Pumphry and S. Rudikoff, unpublished results). We label that subsite as **A** and will show evidence that - when four subsites are labeled **D, B, A** and **C** as shown in Fig. 3-5 across the combining area with the H-chain on the right - the polysaccharide binds with its reducing end projected towards the L chain and that the order of affinities for the subsites is **A > B > C > D**. Two modes of binding for the polysaccharide chain are *a priori* possible (as shown in Figures 3 and 4). We have discussed above that the side of the first galactosyl residue to bind (to subsite **A**) is the face of the pyranosyl ring bearing the 2- and 3-OH groups (41,42,55). The C-6 (the hydroxymethyl group) projects away from the protein toward the solvent as indicated in Figures 3-5. We have also reported that replacement of either the 2- or 3-OH group in methyl β-D-galactopyranoside by fluorine appears to lead to non-binding (49,35, see Table I), which is highly indicative of there being required H-bonding in subsite **A**. It appears from the data (see below) that H-bonding occurs only in subsite A, at least for the 3-OH group of any galactosyl moiety in an oligosaccharide. Fluorine itself does not interfere due to size or charge *per se* when substituting for an OH group (56). Thus, from these data the polysaccharide can be placed in the combining area as shown in either Fig. 3 or Fig. 4. We will show that evidence supports the binding mode shown in Fig. 3 and not that of Fig. 4. Table I lists the maximum changes in the protein tryptophanyl

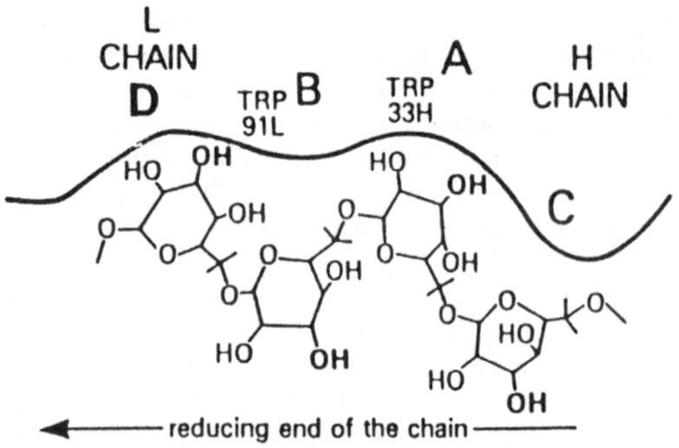

FIGURE 3: Schematic representation of binding mode of a $\beta(1\rightarrow 6)$-D-galactopyranan segment to IgA J539, with the reducing end of the polysaccharide oriented toward the L chain. If the Fc portion of the IgA is called the bottom, the general view is from the top of the protein molecule, looking down along the face of the antibody combining area. The 3-OH groups of each galactosyl residue are boldface. Protein subsites are labeled C, A, B, and D.

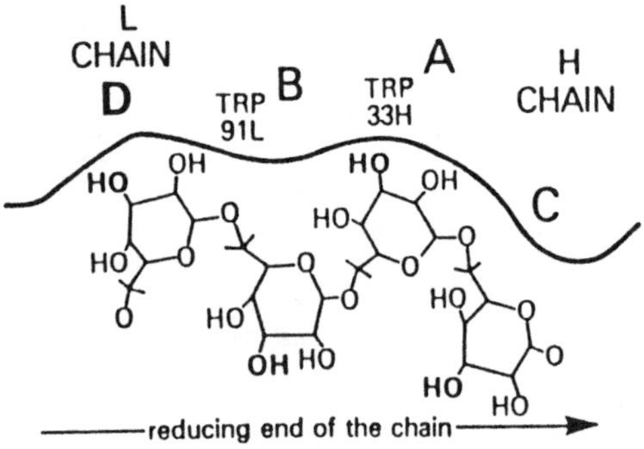

FIGURE 4: Schematic representation of the binding mode of a β-$(1\rightarrow 6)$-D-galactopyranan segment to IgA J539, with the reducing end of the polysaccharide oriented toward the H chain. For other particulars, see legend to Figure 3.

fluorescence (52) induced by a number of our synthetic ligands (a discussion of their preparation will constitute the last part of this article). It can be seen that for the monosaccharides 3-6 this value is ca. 20% (of the total tryptophanyl fluorescence of the antibody). When the ligand increases its length to approximately twice the size, i.e. in going from the monosaccharide methyl β-D-galactopyranoside to 6-O-β-D-galactopyranosyl-D-galactose (Gal$_2$), the value goes up substantially (to 33 %), and even more so for the methyl β-glycoside of Gal$_2$ (7, 36 %) or for the corresponding methyl-Gal$_3$ (10, 43 %). Gal$_2$ has a length of ca. 9 Å. The X-ray diffraction studies of J539 (33) show the two TRP residues 33H and 91L to be ca. 9.5 Å apart. Therefore, the above disaccharide Gal$_2$ with its non-reducing residue in subsite A (and so interfacing the protein

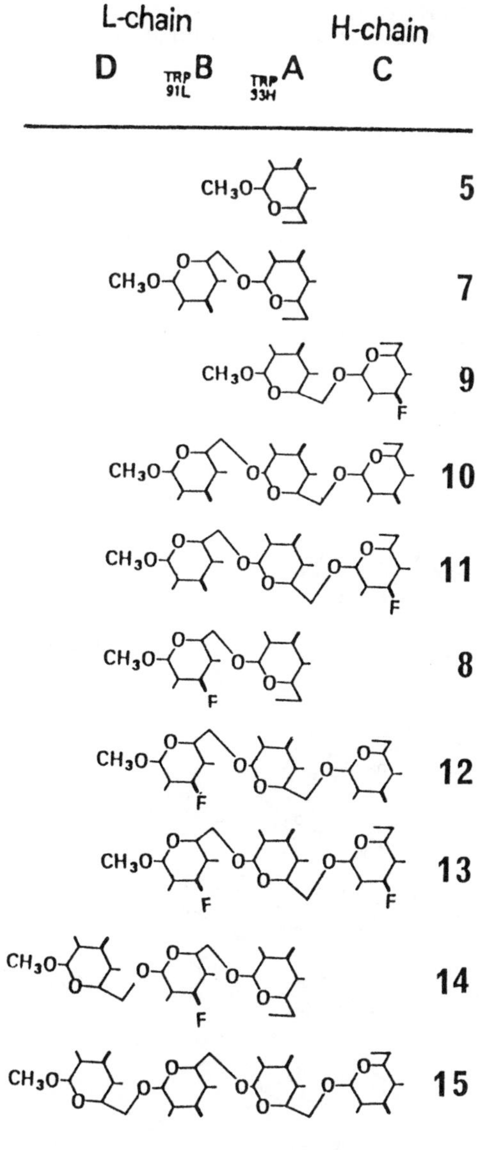

Fig. 5. Schematic representation of the binding of the galactosyl derivatives studied to subsites D, B, A and C.

with its 2- and 3-OH groups), would reach towards TRP 91L with the second galactose unit and perturb that tryptophanyl's fluorscence *only* if in the mode shown in Fig. 3 and not as in Fig. 4. In the latter mode the second galactose residue would project away from the TRP at 91L and would orient more towards

TABLE I BINDING CONSTANTS (K_a) AND MAXIMAL FLUORESCENCE CHANGE (ΔF_{max}) FOR IgA J539 FAB' WITH GALACTOSE DERIVATIVES

	Structure	K_a	ΔF_{max}
1		0	0
2		0	0
3		0.8×10^3	23%
4		2.5×10^3	23%
5		1.0×10^3	21%
6		2.8×10^3	20%
7		4.4×10^4	36%
8		3.7×10^4	45%
9		0.8×10^4	21%
10		4.8×10^5	43%
11		4.1×10^5	42%
12		4.2×10^5	39%
13		3.6×10^5	40%
14		4.2×10^4	41%
15		5.9×10^5	41%
16		5.9×10^5	42%

the H-chain. Thus, the increased maximal fluorescence of the di- and higher $\beta(1\rightarrow6)$-linked galactooligosaccharides supports the binding mode shown in Fig. 3, and we conclude that the reducing end of the polysaccharide antigen projects towards the L chain. Turning to Table I we can interpret the binding data as follows: Methyl galactoside 5 binds at subsite A (see Fig. 5 for a schematic representation). The methyl galactobioside 7 shows a large increase in the maximally induced protein fluorescence, indicating that it is now perturbing both solvent exposed tryptophanyl residues. We therefore place that bioside 7 in subsites A and B (reaching towards the TRP at 91L). Replacing the 3'-OH in 7 with fluorine to obtain 9, brings about a 5-6 times reduction in binding affinity (Table I). It is impossible to accomodate the terminal residue bearing the 3'-deoxy-3'-fluoro group of 9 in subsite A (subsite A requires protein contact with 2- and 3-OH groups). Therefore the methyl deoxy-fluoro bioside 9 shifts to subsite C and A, so that the 2- and 3-OH groups of the methyl galactoside moiety in 9 are instead presented for contact to subsite A in order for 9 to utilize that highest binding subsite. As a result, the 3'-deoxy-3'-fluoro galactosyl group of 9 shifts to subsite C (we will present data later to show that indeed subsite C must be placed next to subsite A and not next to subsite B). If that is correct, the methyl deoxyfluoro galactobioside 9 - unlike the methyl galactobioside 7 - should cause a maximum fluorescence change in the protein like a *mono*saccharide, namely *ca.* 20% (it does not come any nearer the TRP 91L than does 5, and thus only perturbs the TRP 33H near subsite A). Table I shows that this is so. The evidence above suggests an order of affinity for these three subsites as A > B > C. To verify this we measured the affinity of the methyl galactotrioside 10. If the above is correct it must follow that trioside 10 should associate with subsites A, B and C (with an increased affinity compared to that of 7), and that the 3"-deoxy-3"-fluoro derivative of 10, namely 11, should bind with the same affinity as 10. This, because the terminal 3"-deoxy-3"-fluoro-galactosyl group of 11 has its fluorine-bearing galactosyl group bound to subsite C without interference (see Fig. 5). Also, if the trisaccharides 10 and 11 bind in the same subsites A, B and C, they should show the same ligand-induced maximal fluorescence change. The values in Table I show this to be so. Next, the deoxy-fluoro galactobioside 8 was measured. Compound 9 was forced to shift to subsites A and C (see Fig. 5) in order to optimize binding thereby changing the maximal fluorescence change from *ca.* 40% to 20%. Alternatively, saccharide 8 should be capable of binding to subsites A and B with the C2'-C3' face of the terminal galactosyl group hydrogen-bonded in subsite A of the antibody and the 3-deoxy-3-fluoro galactosyl group located in subsite B. Hence its K_a and ΔF_{max} should be the same as that for 7, and Table I bears this out. Similarly, trisaccharides 12 and 13 should be able to bind to subsites B A C, as do 10 and 11 and, again, Table I shows their K_a's and maximal changes in fluorescence to be essentially the same. In order to locate subsite D at either the L or the H chain side of the B A C sequence the trisaccharide 14 was prepared (37). Let us *a priori* place subsite **D** near the L chain. This is reasonable, since if placed near the H chain (next to subsite **C**) it would appear to project too far away from the general antibody combining area. The affinity of **14** for monoclonal IgA J539 Fab' was found to be 4.2 x 10^4 L/M. Since subsite **A** requires interaction of a galactosyl 2- and 3-OH group with the surface of the protein, **14** will be incapable of having its internal D-galactosyl residue engage that subsite, and this trisaccharide can therefore not bind to the **B A C** sequence (see Fig. 5). Assuming the positioning of subsite **D** to be correct, the trisaccharide **14** could bind either to subsite **A C** or to **A B D**, as indicated in Fig. 5. Methyl 6-*O*-(3'-deoxy-3'-fluoro-β-D-galactopyranosyl)-β-D-galactopyranoside (**9**) binds to subsites **A C** with a K_a of 0.8 x 10^4 L/M. Thus, **14**, with a K_a some five times larger must involve additional binding contacts, i.e. subsites **A B D**. Trisaccharide **14** would also have the possibility to bind to *three* subsites if subsite **D** were on the H chain side of subsite **C**. In that case the ΔF_{max} caused by **14** would be expected to be around 20%, since it would then only perturb TRP 33H. However, **14** shows a ΔF_{max} of 40.6% and thus appears to engage TRP 91L. Hence, subsite **D** must be on the L chain side of **B**. This also confirms the **D B A C** arrangement of subsites, rather than **C B A D**, which could have ligand **9** binding to subsites **C B** in that sequence. Such a mode would lower the ΔF_{max} observed, which is associated with the possible perturbation of *one* TRP residue, here residue 91L. However, if that were the case, ligand **14** should have the same K_a as does ligand **10**, and not some ten times less, as observed. (The fact that ligand **11** shows the same K_a and ΔF_{max} as ligand **10** also shows that the subsite sequence **D B A C** is correct and not the sequence **C B A D**). The above observations on the location of subsite **D** also agree with the finding that the K_a found for **14** (4.2 x 10^4 L/M) is only sligthly higher than the previously reported K_a for ligand **8** (3.6 x 10^4). This reflects only a small additional binding due to subsite **D**. We have shown that the maximally binding methyl β-glycoside of β(1→6)-linked D-galactotetraose (**15**) binds (39) to IgA J539 Fab' with a K_a of 0.59 x 10^6 L/M, while the corresponding trioside **10** binds with a K_a of 0.48 x 10^6 L/M, revealing the small additional binding of the fourth subsite. Lastly, note (Table I) that **4** shows a significant increase in binding compared to **5**. This does *not* appear to be due to H-bond acceptance by the 6-position, since compound **6**, lacking the 6-OH group, shows an identical increase in binding. We have no explanation for this observation.

Having thus established the likely arrangement of galactosyl binding subsites in IgA J539, we turn our attention to other members of the β(1→6)-D-galactopyranan binding monoclonal antibodies. Potter *et al.* (43) and our laboratory (14,57) have over the years identified many individual myeloma and hybridoma monoclonal antibodies with this specificity. It is important to see if all these anti-galactan immunoglobulins, whose amino acid sequence we know, show similar or dissimilar subsite arrangements. Thus, it may be possible to propose or dismiss certain amino acid residues responsible for bonding to the ligand by comparing the sequences occuring in the hypervariable regions.

In Table II are listed the constants of association (K_a) of compounds **2**, **5**, **7-11**, **15** and **16** with seven monoclonal anti-$\beta(1{\rightarrow}6)$-D-galactopyranans, as well as the maximal fluorescence changes of these proteins on binding the ligand in question (58). These seven antibodies all belong to the same family (44) and their amino acid sequence is known (28,34,43). From the K_a values of **5** , **7**, **10**, **15**, and **16** with IgA (Fab') J539 it can be deduced that the four subsites **C**, **A**, **B** and **D** have vastly different affinities for "their" individual galactosyl residue, namely 10^3 (**A**), 47 (**B**), 10 (**C**) and 1.3 (**D**), and thus only subsite **A** has a high affinity. It is interesting that that highest binding subsite is located *internally* in the sequence of subsites (59). It can also be learned from Table II that all anti-galactan antibodies show the same K_a pattern: methyl 3-deoxy-3-fluoro-β-D-galactopyranoside (**2**) shows no noticable binding, while methyl β-D-galactopyranoside (**5**) shows *relatively* the strongest binding (as $-\triangle G$/sugar residue) when compared to methyl O-β-D-galactopyranosyl-(1→6)-β-D-galactopyranoside (**7**) and the corresponding tri- (**10**), tetra- (**15**) and pentasachharide (**16**). That is to say, for ligands **5**, **7**, **10**, **15** and **16** the $\triangle G$ ($\triangle G$ = -RTlnK$_a$) of binding are such that the - $\triangle G$ for **5** is the highest *per sugar residue*. Therefore, all these antibodies posess one galactosyl-binding subsite having an affinity for "its" sugar residue which far exceeds the affinities which the other three subsites have for their galactosyl residues. Methyl O-3-deoxy-3-fluoro-β-D-galactopyranosyl-(1→6)-β-D-galactopyranoside (**9**) binds substantially less than the nonfluorinated disaccharide **7**, whereas the isomeric disaccharide **8** binds to the proteins studied with similar K_a's as does **7**. As we pointed out above, this is due to the fact that **7** binds to the two subsites with the highest affinities (**A** and **B**) whereas **9** must shift to the subsites **A** and **C** in order to be able to use the two required hydrogen-bonding hydroxyl groups demanded by subsite **A**. Again, in so doing ligand **9** should then only perturb the TRP at position 33H, and it can be seen in Table II that its maximal fluorescence change is less than that for **7** in all cases except for IgA X44 (for an explanation see below). Ligand **8** can again bind to subsites **A** and **B**, and thus will show essentially the same K_a and F_{max} as does **7**. This pattern holds for all the antibodies studied here (for IgA X44 the F_{max} stays the same, see below). All this is consistent with the same subsite arrangement for all of these antibodies. In all cases, except for hybridoma HyG 1 (lack of antibody supply), this was moreover confirmed by comparison of the K_a and F_{max} values for the trioside **10** with those for methyl O-3-deoxy-3-fluoro-β-D-galactopyranosyl-(1→6)-O-β-D-galactopyranosyl-(1→6)-β-D-galactopyranoside (**11**), which should be, and are, very similar. Therefore, the way in which these ligands contact the antibodies involved appears to be the same in all cases.

Table III lists the known (28,34,43) amino acid sequences for the variable parts of the H and L chains of the seven antibodies studied. Kabat *et al.* (38) have tabulated the known amino acid sequences of immunoglobulins. In there the sequences

TABLE II. Binding constants, K_a, and percentage maximal fluorescence change (ΔF_{max}, in parentheses) for monoclonal immunoglobulins with galactose derivatives

Compound		Immunoglobulin						
		X-44	J539	X-24	T601	HyG-10	HyG-1	S-10
5		0.4×10^3 (-9)	1.0×10^3 (+21)	0.5×10^3 (+21)	0.4×10^3 (+15)	0.7×10^3 (+26)	1.3×10^3 (+10)	– (-3)
7		1.9×10^4 (-8)	4.7×10^4 (+41)	2.1×10^4 (+35)	1.3×10^4 (+30)	3.1×10^4 (+41)	1.6×10^4 (+21)	2.0×10^4 (+9)
10		2.1×10^5 (-11)	4.8×10^5 (+43)	3.2×10^5 (+41)	2.6×10^5 (+31)	2.1×10^5 (+41)	–	1.0×10^5 (+9)
15		3.2×10^5 (-9)	5.9×10^5 (+41)	5.7×10^5 (+40)	3.2×10^5 (+32)	3.2×10^5 (+43)	1.8×10^5 (+20)	2.1×10^5 (+12)
16		3.2×10^5 (-9)	5.9×10^5 (+42)	6.2×10^5 (+40)	–	3.9×10^5 (+42)	3.1×10^5 (+18)	2.0×10^5 (+10)
8		3.3×10^4 (-7)	3.7×10^4 (+45)	1.7×10^4 (+38)	1.5×10^4 (+31)	3.1×10^4 (+46)	1.6×10^4 (+19)	2.6×10^4 (+10)
9		4.1×10^3 (-11)	7.0×10^3 (+23)	6.3×10^3 (+20)	4.0×10^3 (+15)	3.0×10^3 (+24)	2.2×10^3 (+9)	– (-2)
11		1.6×10^5 (-9)	4.1×10^5 (+42)	3.0×10^5 (+38)	2.1×10^5 (+31)	1.5×10^5 (+42)	–	1.0×10^5 (+9)
2		0	0	0	0	0	0	0

TABLE III. H-chain V-region sequences of murine BALB/c galactan-binding monoclonal immunoglobulins

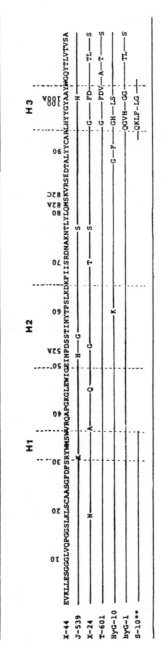

L-chain V-region sequences of murine BALB/c galactan-binding monoclonal immunoglobulins

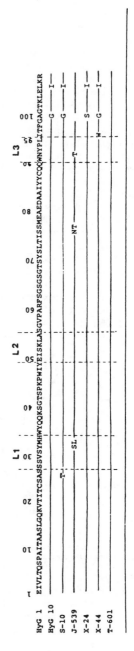

of some 51 monoclonal immunoglobulins of varied specificities
(anti-phosphorylcholine, -2,1-fructan, 2,6-fructan, -dextran, -β-
N-acetyl-glucosaminyl, -galactan) and having H chains belonging
to sub-group III have been listed. Some twenty others have been
partly sequenced to residue 36. It is interesting that - with the
exception of IgG MOPC 173 having no known specificity - only the
anti-carbohydrate immunoglobulins have a TRP at position 33H (and
we have found that MOPC 173 is "related" to anti-2,6-fructan, and
thus to an anti-carbohydrate, see ref. 60). Of these sequenced
antibodies, only the anti-fructans and the anti-galactans show an
asparagine (ASN) at position 58H in addition to the TRP at 33H.
Of some 85 monoclonal murine kappa L chains which have been
completely sequenced, only the anti-galactans (and three other
immunoglobulins of as yet unknown specificity) have a TRP at
position 91L and a proline (PRO) at position 94L. It can be seen
from the X-ray data (33) that ASN 58H, TRP 33H and PRO 94L are
clustered together with the Cα distance for PRO 94L - ASN 58H
around 7 Å and the distance of the Cα's of that PRO and ASN to
the TRP 33H ring system from 9-13 Å and 7-11 Å respectively (see
stereo Fig. 6). The subsite with the highest galactosyl-binding
affinity appears near the H chain, and it is quite possible that
the above three residues make up this subsite. In addition,
certain differing amino acids in the second hypervariable region
of the heavy chain (in Table III referred to as H2) may be
eliminated as likely candidates for direct hydrogen-bonding to
the (poly)saccharide: histidine 52H (this confirms our earlier
work, see ref. 61) in J539, aspartic acid 53H in X44, J539, T601,
HyG10 and HyG1, serine 55H in all (J539 has a glycine at that

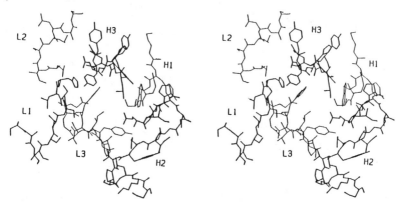

Fig. 6. The complementarity determining regions (CDRs) of IgA J539 according to Suh *et al.* (33).
Alternating CDRs are drawn lightly and boldly. The TRP (33H), ASN (58H) and PRO (94L) in the right
lower quadrant are clearly visible.

position) and threonine 60H in all but HyG 10, which has a lysine
there. Also, from Table III it can be seen that the the third
hypervariable region in these antibodies show much variation in
sequence. Since binding behaviour is so similar, it appears that
the contribution to binding by this epitope can be ignored.
Lastly, it can be seen in Table II that X44 has an unusual ligand

induced fluorescence behaviour, in that the change is essentially invariant with the size of the ligand in contrast to the other antibodies. Visual examination of the crystal structure of J539 (Fab') (33) shows that the TRP 91L, although turned towards the protein, is situated as part of the wall of the frontal cavity, and thus appears perturbable. It can be seen that IgA X44 is the only protein in this group which has an additional TRP at position 96L instead of an isoleucine (ILEU). Examination of the hv_L-3 loop of J539 in the X-ray structure (33) shows that position 96L is relatively close to position 91L. X44 may have a three-dimensional structure which is relatively close to that of J539. If so, may it be possible that in X44 these two tryptophan residues are stacked so that the energy can transfer between them? If so the TRP 91L in X44 may not be easily perturbable by ligands.

PREPARATION OF LIGANDS OF THE β-D-*GALACTO* SERIES
Our preparation of the many methyl β-glycosides of β-(1→6)-D-galacto-oligosaccharides - some of which carried one or more deoxyfluoro groups - was instrumental in the elucidation of binding modes described above. The latter were concerned more with the binding contribution of the *immunoglobulin* than with the contribution of the *ligand*. This laboratory had shown earlier (40-42,49,55,59) the areas of importance to binding occurring on the ligand. Synthetic procedures associated with that earlier work will not be reviewed here. We here describe our approach to the syntheses of derivatives of 1) deoxyfluoro derivatives of methyl β-D-galactopyranoside, as well as 2) methyl β-glycosides of (1→6)-β-D-galacto-oligosaccharides and their specifically fluorinated analogs.

In our initial studies (40, 41) reducing oligosaccharides had been used. However, methyl β-glycosides more closely imitate the situation in the polymeric antigen, (1→6)-β-D-galactopyranan (39), and all our oligo- and deoxyfluoro-oligosaccharides, prepared since, were methyl β-glycosides.

Monodeoxyfluoro derivatives of methyl β-D-galactopyranoside were synthesized by the introduction of fluorine at specific positions. Certain hydroxyl groups in a sugar derivative (not necessarily having a D-*galacto* configuration) were blocked to arrive at a precursor suitable for a C-OH → C-F conversion. The only exception to direct C-OH → C-F transformation was the introduction of fluorine *via* D-galactal, using xenon difluoride, leading (49) to **1** (Scheme 1).

To effect other fluorinations, we have used a number of reagents ranging from a common source of fluoride ion such as cesium fluoride (62) to one such as polymer-bound fluoride (A-26-F, ion exchange resin). Using the latter reagent, we have been able to improve (49,62,63) the yield (64) of methyl 4-deoxy-4-fluoro-β-D-galactopyranoside (**3**), obtained after deblocking of its 2,3-di-*O*-benzyl-6-*O*-trityl derivative (Scheme 2). The most versatile fluorinating reagents, now available for the replacement of a hydroxyl group for fluorine, seem to be diethylaminosulfur trifluoride (DAST) and its methyl analog

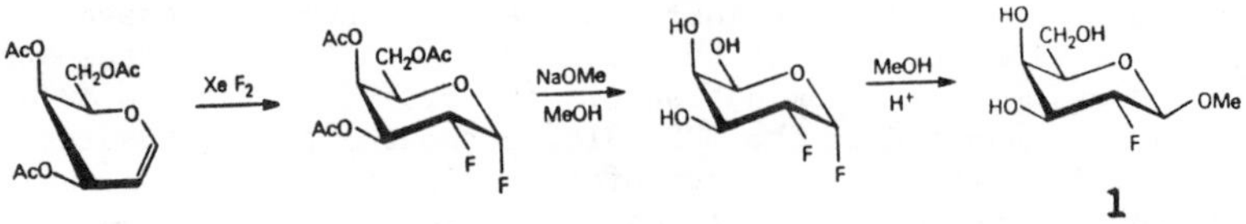

Scheme 1

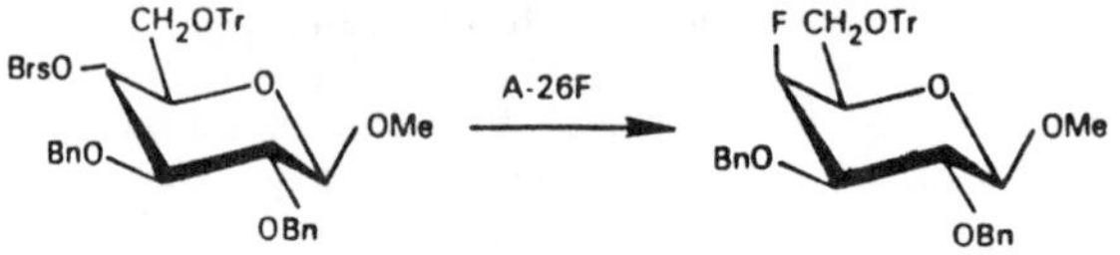

Scheme 2

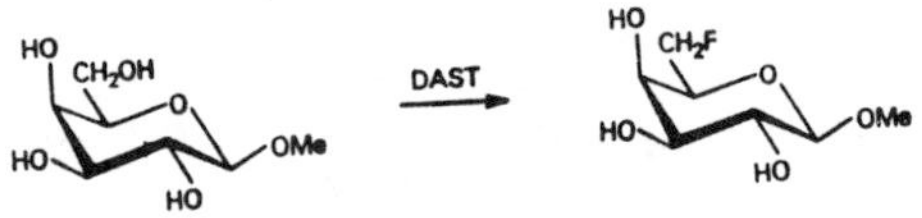

Scheme 3

(methyl DAST, 65). We used DAST to prepare (Scheme 3) methyl 6-deoxy-6-fluoro-β-D-galactopyranoside (**4**, 63), as well as its 3-fluoro analog (**2**, 62). DAST was especially useful in the preparation of the latter derivative (Scheme 4). Fluorination with inversion of configuration of position 3 of the D-gulose derivative **17**, prepared from D-glucose, as shown below, could be markedly improved in comparison to fluorinations mediated by tetraethylammonium bromide or by an ion exchange resin in the fluoride form.

After it had become apparent that hydrogen bonding involving hydroxyl groups at positions 2 (ref. 49) and 3 (ref. 62) in D-galactose play an important role in binding of the carbohydrate to antigalactan monoclonal immunoglobulins, our next task was to obtain deoxyfluoro ligands closely related to the (1→6)-β-D-galactopyranan antigen. From the studies involving monodeoxyfluoro derivatives of methyl β-D-galactopyranoside, we knew that replacement of either the 2-OH or 3-OH group by fluorine causes cessation of binding to the highest binding antibody subsite **A** (35,49). Thus, if the modified oligo-saccharides would contain a 2- or 3-deoxyfluoro-D-galactose at a certain position (or positions) in the oligosaccharide sequence, it would force that galactosyl moiety not to bind to the subsite **A**. Clearly, only the use of 3-deoxy-3-fluoro-D-galactopyranosyl halide derivatives would allow us to use a 2-O-acyl group as a blocking moiety. This, in turn, through its anchimeric trans-directing action, would stereoselectively result in the formation of the desired β-galactosidic linkage. The useful starting

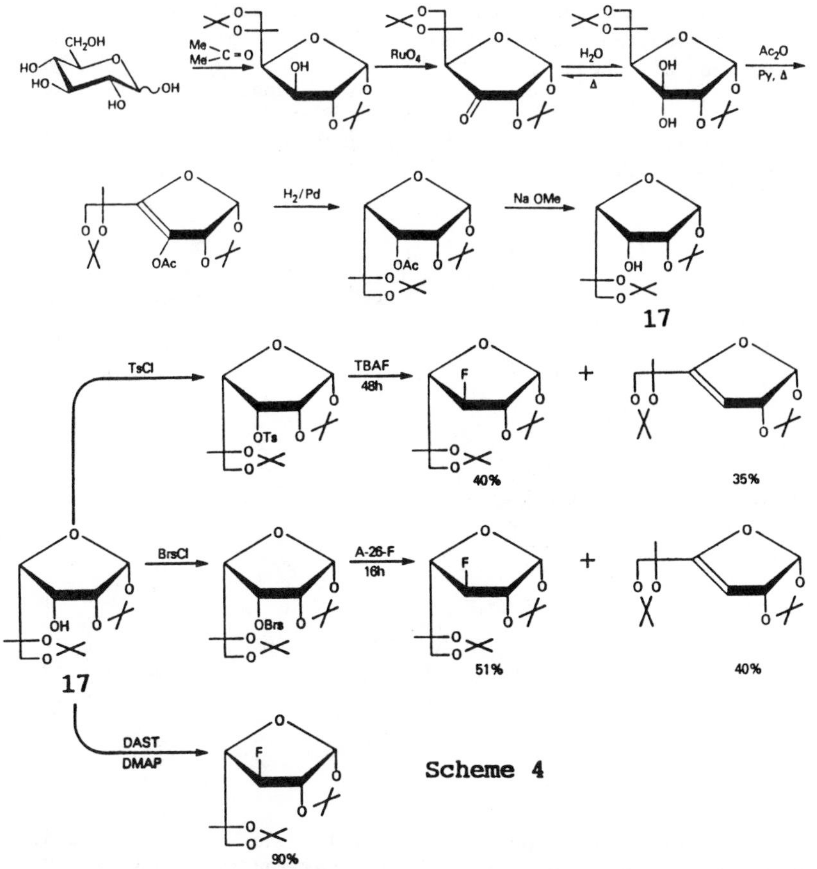

Scheme 4

material for the synthesis of such a halide appeared to be a 2,4,6-tri-O-acyl-3-deoxy-3-fluoro-α- or -β-D-galactopyranose. Acetylation of 3-deoxy-3-fluoro-D-galactose with acetic anhydride in the presence of sodium acetate at an elevated temperature, conditions under which β-1-O-acetyl derivatives are often formed in high yields, had been previously described. However, the reported low yield (35%, 66) of the only pyranosyl isomer isolated, crystalline β-1-O-acetate, was due to extensive formation of acetates having the furanose structure. Clearly, a prerequisite of an *efficient* conversion to a halide such as **19** is finding reaction conditions for the acetylation of 3-deoxy-3-fluoro-D-galactose whereby the combined yield of **18α** and **18β** would be high. This we realized (Scheme 5) when acetylation of 3-deoxy-3-fluoro-D-galactose with acetic anhydride in pyridine was conducted initially at subzero temperature. That the formation of acetyl derivatives having furanose structure was minimal can be deduced from the observed high yield of crystalline **19**.

Construction of methyl β-glycosides of (1→6)-β-D-galacto-oligosaccharides followed the strategy developed earlier in this laboratory (67). Accordingly, a selectively removable (haloacetyl) group was used for the temporary protection of position 6 in the D-galactosyl halides employed for the construction of these oligosaccharides. Such a halide has to have, in addition, a group at position 2 capable of anchimeric assistance in replacing the leaving group at C-1. Originally, we used 2,3,4-tri-O-acetyl-6-O-(chloroacetyl)-α-D-galactopyranosyl bromide (**20**, ref. 67). In this way, the methyl β-glycosides

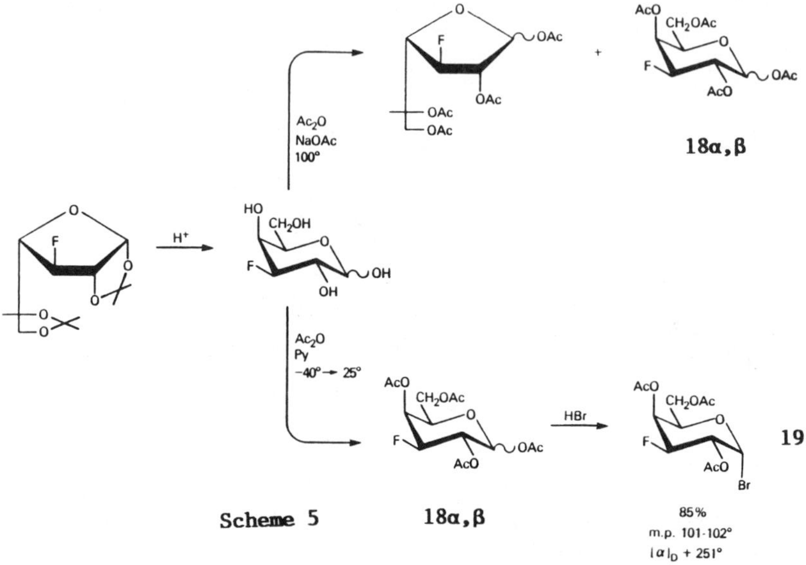

Scheme 5   18α,β

of(1→6)-β-linked D-galactotriose (**10**) and the related, fluorinated trisaccharide **11** were synthesized (68). However, we observed that noticeable migration of acetyl groups occurred during de(chloroacetyl)ation of intermediates with thiourea. Hydroxyl groups protected with the bromoacetyl group can be regenerated under much milder conditions than those protected with the chloroacetyl groups. Therefore, to construct (69)

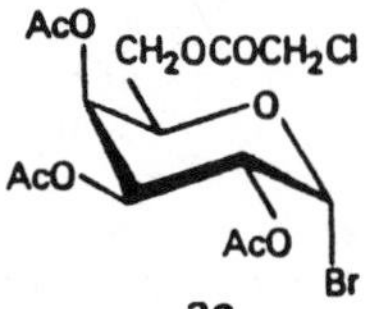

20

internal units of the fluorinated oligosaccharides **12** and **21** 2,3,4-tri-O-acetyl-6-O-(bromoacetyl)-α-D-galactopyranosyl bromide (**22**, 69) was used as the glycosyl donor (Scheme 6). Acetyl group migration during de(haloacetyl)ation could be minimized in this way. However, formation of by-products, mainly O-acetyl derivatives of the employed nucleophiles (70), during

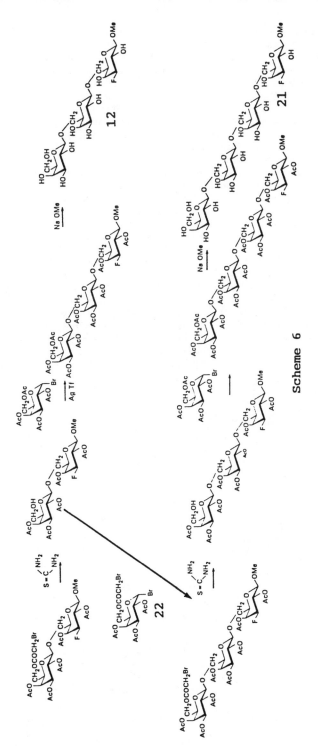

Scheme 6

glycosylations promoted by silver trifluoromethanesulfonate could still not be entirely overcome when *O*-acetylated reactants were used. Therefore, in subsequent syntheses of methyl β-glycosides of (1→6)-β-D-galacto-oligosaccharides, and their specifically fluorinated analogs, *benzoylated* intermediates were used. The strategy of using the bromoacetyl group for the temporary protection of position 6 in otherwise fully benzoylated derivatives of D-galactose required the preparation of a large number of variously substituted intermediates. For example (Fig. 7), the specifically fluorinated trisaccharide **13** contains 3-deoxy-3-fluoro-D-galactose in both end-units, and its synthesis requires two different derivatives of 3-deoxy-3-fluoro-D-galactose as intermediates. In addition, to form the internal unit of the trisaccharide, a complex glycosyl donor derived from D-galactose is required. Such a synthon, 2,3,4-tri-*O*-benzoyl-6-*O*-bromoacetyl-α-D-galactopyranosyl bromide (**23**, Scheme 7), was prepared (71) from D-galactose *via* either of the two tetra-*O*-benzoyl derivatives **24** or **25** (only the route involving **24** is shown). 2,4-6-Tri-*O*-benzoyl-3-deoxy-3-fluoro-α-D-galacto-pyranosyl bromide (**26**), used to construct the glycosyl end-group of the oligosaccharide (Fig. 7), was prepared (71) from 3-deoxy-3-fluoro-D-galactose as shown in Scheme 8. Referring to Fig. 7, methyl 2,4-di-*O*-benzoyl-3-deoxy-3-fluoro-β-D-galactopyranoside (shown at the bottom right of Fig. 7) was condensed with a fully blocked galactosyl halide (**23**) bearing a group at *O*-6 which could be removed selectively. Subsequent removal of that group, followed by condensation of the product with the deoxyfluoro

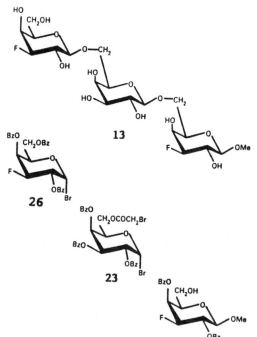

Figure 7. Specifically fluorinated trisaccharide **13** containing 3-deoxy-3-fluoro-D-galactose in both end-units.

galactosyl halide (**26**), followed by complete deblocking, then yielded **13**. The synthesis of the closely related trisaccharide **14** required different intermediates.   Synthesis of its fully benzoylated precursor is shown in Scheme 9. The key intermediate used to form the internal 3-deoxy-3-fluoro-β-D-galactopyranosyl residue of the oligosaccharide, 2,4-di-*O*-benzoyl-6-*O*-bromoacetyl-3-deoxy-3-fluoro-α-D-galactopyranosyl chloride (**27**), was obtained (37) from the corresponding methyl β-glycoside by cleavage (72) with dichloromethyl methyl ether (DCMME)/ZnCl$_2$ reagent.

Glycosyl bromide **23** proved to be an excellent glycosyl donor, but its large-scale preparation, required for the stepwise construction of higher (1→6)-linked β-D-galacto-oligosaccharides or their methyl glycosides, is somewhat tedious (Scheme 7). It requires isolation of all intermediates by chromatography, involving, *inter alia,* the separation of four isomeric tetra-*O*-benzoyl-D-galactoses, to remove from the crude product the

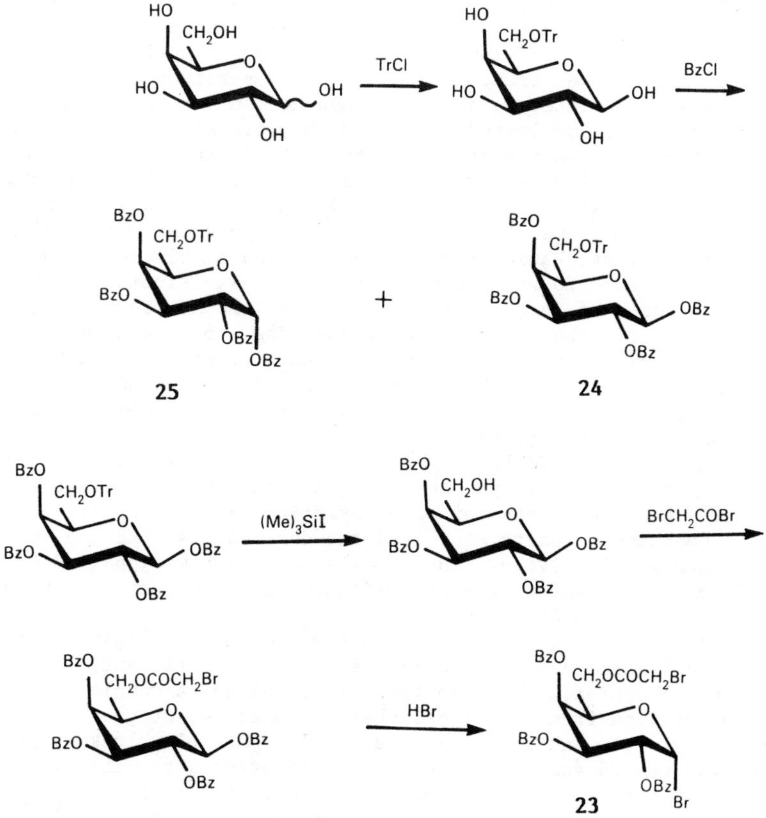

Scheme 7

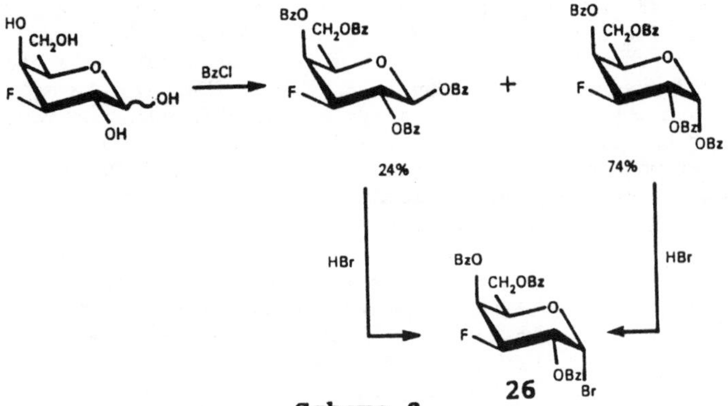

Scheme 8

furanose isomers formed during the benzoylation of 6-O-trityl-D-galactose. Therefore, a more efficient source of a suitable glycosylating reagent related to **23** was sought. To prevent the formation of 5-membered ring forms during synthetic manipulations, we changed the synthetic strategy and decided to use as a key intermediate a compound in which the pyranose structure would be locked before further transformations would be attempted. These requirements are met in an excellent way by methyl 2,3,4-tri-O-benzoyl-β-D-galactopyranoside (**28**), a readily obtainable crystalline compound (73), which we used as a pivotal intermediate to synthesize methyl β-glycosides of (1→6)-β-D-galacto-oligosaccharides by a stepwise and a blockwise approach (74). Compound **28** was used firstly, in a way similar to that in the synthesis of **14** (c.f. Scheme 9), as the nucleophile in the syntheses of the said oligosaccharides, up to and including a hexasaccharide. Secondly, it was the key intermediate in the preparation of 2,3,4-tri-O-benzoyl-6-O-(bromoacetyl)-α-D-galactopyranosyl chloride (**29**). Thus, (Scheme 10) compound **28** was (bromoacetyl)ated and the resulting 6-O-(bromoacetyl) derivative was cleaved with DCMME/ZnCl$_2$ to yield (84%) the glycosyl chloride **29**. Crystalline glycosyl chloride **29** is sufficiently reactive under the conditions of glycosylation promoted by silver tri-fluoromethanesulfonate, to yield the desired disaccharide **30** with high stereoselectivity. The stepwise approach was applied to the synthesis of lower oligosaccharides in this series, as shown in Scheme 11.

To obtain the higher members of methyl β-glycosides of (1→6)-β-D-galacto-oligosaccharides a more efficient, blockwise synthetic approach was applied. It required a complex glycosyl donor derived from an oligosaccharide, bearing at position 6 of its glycosyl end-group a selectively removable blocking group. Derivatives **24** and **25**, isolated in connection with the synthesis of **23** (Scheme 7), were used as intermediates in the preparation of such a glycosyl donor (**31**). As shown in Scheme 12, **24** and **25** were each detritylated and then condensed with the

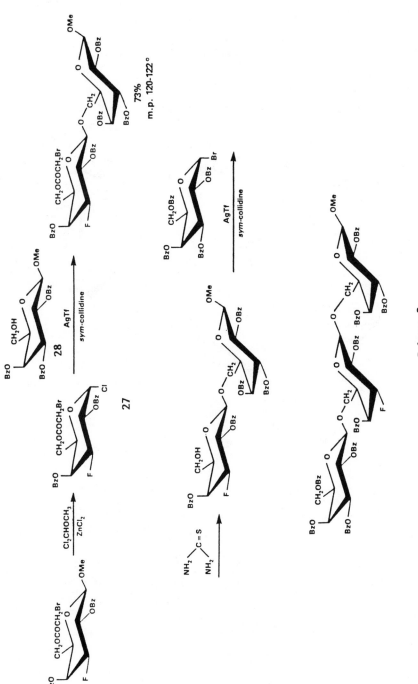

Scheme 9

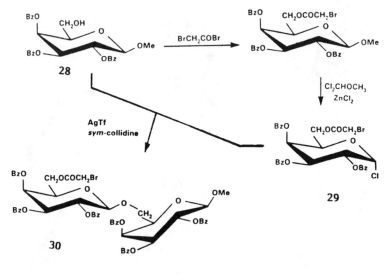

Scheme 10

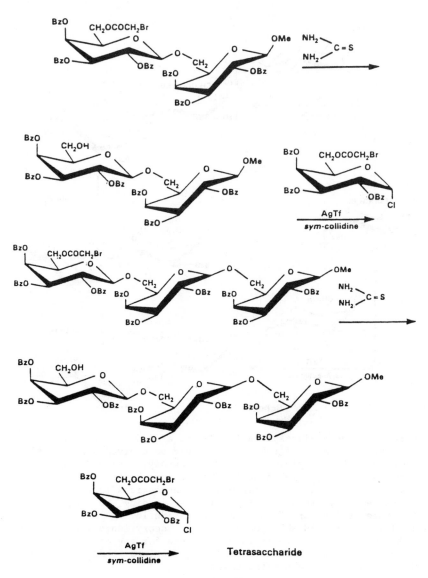

Scheme 11

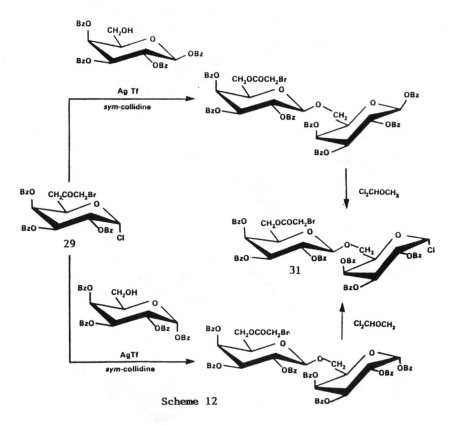

Scheme 12

(bromoacetyl)ated glycosyl halide **29**, to afford the corresponding disaccharides. Each of the latter could be cleaved subsequently with DCMME/ZnCl$_2$ to yield the same glycosyl chloride (**31**), a derivative of (1→6)-β-linked galactobiose. Its use in the blockwise synthesis of the target oligosaccharides is exemplified in Scheme 13, showing the pathway leading to the fully substituted precursor of the pentasaccharide **16**.

Finally, from the ^{1}H NMR spectra of our deoxyfluoro ligands, it has become clear that there is *no* evidence for any conformational change due to the introduction of fluorine into these molecules (cf. ref. 37 and papers cited therein).

CONCLUSION

This review shows the application of the combination of bromoacetyl and benzoyl groups, as temporary and permanent blocking groups in oligosaccharide synthesis. In this way, we have been able to prepare systematically, and with a high degree of stereoselecivity, specifically fluorinated ligands for anti-galactan monoclonal immunoglobulins. Next, our work has shown the extraordinary usefulness of these deoxyfluoro (oligo)saccharides in unraveling *details* of the binding of these monoclonal antibodies to their carbohydrate antigens.

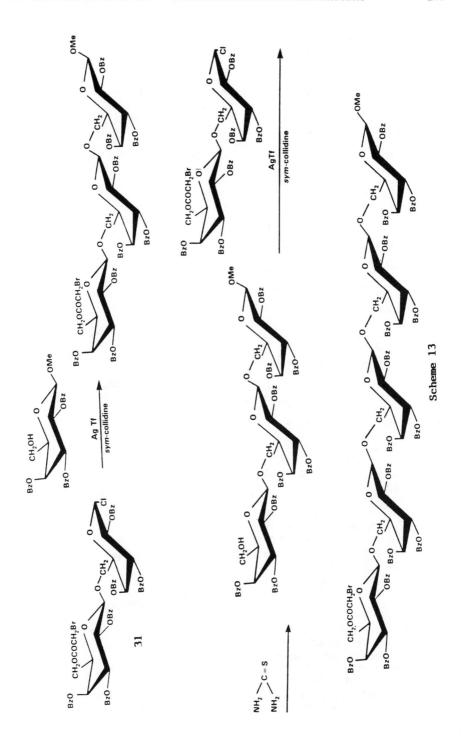

Scheme 13

Literature Cited

1. Burnet, F. M. *The Clonal Selection of Acquired Immunity*. Van der Bilt University Press, Nashville, Tenn, 1959.
2. Klinman, N. R. *J. Exp. Med.* 1972, **136**, 241.
3. Graeves, M.; Janossy, G. *Transpl. Rev.* 1972, **11**, 87.
4. Krause, R. M. *Adv. Immunol.* 1971, **12**, 1.
5. Haber, E. *Ann. N. Y. Acad. Sci.* 1972, **190**, 283.
6. Potter, M. In *Cancer: A Comprehensive Treatise*, Becker, F. F., Ed.: Plenum, N. Y. 1975, **1**, 161.
7. Potter, M.; Glaudemans, C. P. J. *Methods Enzymol.* 1972, **28**, 388.
8. Warner, N. L. *Immunogenetics* 1975, **2**, 1.
9. Cohn, M. *Cold Spring Harbor Symp. Quant. Biol.* 1967, **32**, 211.
10. Eisen, H. N.; Simms, E. S.; Potter, M. *Biochem.* 1968, **7**, 4126.
11. Potter, M.; Leon, M. A. *Science* 1968, **162**, 369.
12. Melchers, F.; Potter, M.; Warner, N. Eds. *Lymphocyte Hybridomas*: Springer Verlag 1979.
13. Köhler, G.; Milstein C. *Nature* 1975, **256**, 495.
14. Glaudemans, C. P. J.; Das, M. K.; Vrana, M. *Methods Enzymol.* 1978, **50**, 316.
15. Kabat, E. A. *Pharm. Rev.* 1982, **34**, 23.
16. Glaudemans, C. P. J. *Adv. Carbohydr. Chem. Biochem.* 1975, **31**, 313.
17. Padlan, E. A.; Segal, D. M.; Spande, T. F.; Davies, D. R.; Rudikoff, S.; Potter, M. *Nature* 1973, **145**, 165.
18. Poljak, R. J.; Amzel, L. M.; Avey, H. P.; Chen. B. L.; Phizakerley, R. P.,; Saul, F. *Proc. Nat. Acad. Sci. U.S.A.* 1973, **70**, 3305.
19. Segal, D. M.; Padlan, E. A.; Cohen, G. H.; Rudikoff, S.; Potter, M; Davies, D. R. *Proc. Nat. Acad. Sci. U.S.A.* 1974, **71**, 4298.
20. Sciffer, M.; Girling, R. L.; Ely, K. R.; Edmundson, A. B. *Biochem.* 1973, **12**, 4620.
21. Epp, O.; Colman, P.; Fehlhammer, H.; Bode, W.; Schiffer, M.; Huber, R.; Palm, W. *Eur. J. Biochem.* 1974, **45**, 513.
22. Padlan, E. A. *Quart. Rev. Biophys.* 1977, **10**, 35.
23. Porter, R. R. *Harvey Lect.* 1971, **65**, 157.
24. Wu, T. T.; Kabat, E. A. *J. Exp. Med.* 1970, **132**, 211.
25. Rudikoff, S. In *Contemporary Topics in Molecular Immunology* 1983, **9** 169.
26. Seydman, J. G.; Maxx, E. E.; Leder, P. *Proc. Nat. Acad. Sci. U.S.A.*, **76**, 3450.
27. Early, P.; Huang, H.; Davis, M.; Calame, K.; Hood, L. *Cell* 1980, **19**, 981.
28. Rudikoff, S.; Rao, N. D.; Glaudemans, C. P. J.; Potter, M. *Proc. Nat. Acad. Sci. U.S.A.* 1980, **77**, 4270.
29. Potter, M. *Adv. Immunol.* 1977, **25**, 141.
30. Gearhart, P. J.; Johnson, N. D.; Douglas, R.; Hood, L. *Nature* 1981, **291**, 29.
31. Andres, C. M.; Maddelena, A.; Hudak, S.; Young, N. M.; Claflin, J. L. *J. Exp. Med.* 1981, **154**, 1570.

32. Satow, Y.; Cohen, G. H.; Padlan, E. A.; Davies, D. R. *J. Mol. Biol.* 1986, **190**, 593.
33. Suh, S. W.; Bhat, T. N.; Navia, M. A.; Cohen, G. H.; Rao, D. N.; Rudikoff, S.; Davies, D. R. *Proteins: Structure, Function and Genetics* 1986, **1**, 74.
34. Pawlita, M.; Potter, M.; Rudikoff, S. *J. Immunol.* 1982, **129**, 615.
35. Glaudemans, C. P. J.; Kováč, P.; Rasmussen, K. *Biochem.* 1984, **23**, 6732.
36. Glaudemans, C. P. J.; Kováč, P. *Mol. Immunol.* 1985, **22**, 651.
37. Kováč, P.; Glaudemans, C. P. J. *J. Carbohydr. Chem.* 1986, **4**, 613.
38. Kabat, E. A.; Wu, T. T.; Bilofsky, H.; Reid-Miller, M.; Perry, M.; Gottesman, K. *Sequences of Proteins of Immunological Interest.* U.S. Dept. of H.H.S., P.H.S., N.I.H., Bethesda, MD, U.S.A. 1987.
39. Glaudemans, C. P. J.; Bhattacharjee, A. K.; Manjula, B. N. *Molec. Immunol.* 1986, **23**, 655.
40. Jolley, M. E.; Rudikoff, S.; Potter, M.; Glaudemans, C. P. J. *Biochem.* 1973, **12**, 3039.
41. Jolley, M. E.; Glaudemans, C. P. J.; Rudikoff, S.; Potter, M. *Biochem.* 1974, **13**, 3179.
42. Ekborg, G.; Ittah, Y.; Glaudemans, C. P. J. *Molec. Immunol.* 1983, **20**, 235.
43. Rudikoff, S.; Pawlita, M.; Pumphry, J.; Mushinsky, E. B.; Potter, M. *J. Exp. Med.* 1983, **158**, 1385.
44. Hartman, A. B.; Rudikoff, S. *EMBO J.* 1984, **3**, 3023.
45. Ekborg, G.; Vranešić, B.; Bhattacharjee, A. K.; Kováč, P.; Glaudemans, C. P. J. *Carbohydr. Res.* 1985, **143**, 203.
46. Falent-Kwast, E.M.; Kováč, P.; Bax, A.; Glaudemans, C. P. J. *Carbohydr. Res.* 1986, **145**, 332.
47. Nashed, E. M.; Glaudemans, C. P. J. *Carbohydr. Res.* 1986, **158**, 125.
48. Jung, G. L.; Holme, K. R.; Glaudemans, C. P. J.; Lehmann, J.; Lay, H. *Carbohydr. Res.* ms. submitted.
49. Ittah, Y.; Glaudemans, C. P. J. *Carbohydr. Res.* 1981, **95**, 189.
50. Goldstein, I. J.; Hayes, C. E. *Adv. Carbohydr. Chem.Biochem.* 1978, **35**, 127, and references therein.
51. Lemieux, R. U.; Bock, K. *Arch. Biochem. Biophys.* 1983, **221**, 125.
52. Jolley, M. E.; Glaudemans, C. P. J. *Carbohydr. Res.* 1974, **33**, 377.
53. Rao, D. N.; Rudikoff, S.; Krutzsch, H.; Potter, M. *Proc. Nat. Acad. Sci. U.S.A.* 1979, **76**, 2890.
54. Manjula, B. N.; Mushinski, E. B.; Glaudemans, C. P. J. *J. Immunol.* 1979, **119**, 867.
55. Glaudemans, C. P. J.; Zissis, E.; Jolley, M. E. *Carbohydr. Res.* 1975, **40**, 129.
56. Murray-Rust, P.; Stallings, W. C.; Monti, C. T.; Preston, R. K.; Glusker, J. P. *J. Amer. Chem. Soc.* 1983, **105**, 3206.
57. Manjula, B. N.; Glaudemans, C. P. J.; Mushinsky, E. B.; Potter, M. *Carbohydr. Res.* 1975, **40**, 37.
58. Glaudemans, C. P. J. *Mol. Immunol.* 1987, **24**, 371.

59. Glaudemans, C. P. J. *Mol. Immunol.* 1986, **23**, 917.
60. Enghofer, E.; Glaudemans, C. P. J.; Bosma, M. J. *Molec. Immunol.* 1979, **16**, 1103.
61. Gettings, P.; Boyd, J.; Glaudemans, C. P. J.; Potter, M.; Dwek, R. A. *Biochem.* 1981, **20**, 7463.
62. Kováč, P.; Glaudemans, C. P. J. *Carbohydr. Res.* 1983, **123**, 326.
63. Kováč, P.; Glaudemans, C. P. J. J. *Carbohydr. Chem.* 1983, **2**, 313.
64. Maradufu, A.; Perlin, A. S. *Carbohydr. Res.* 1974, **32**, 261.
65. Kováč, P.; Sklenar, V.; Glaudemans, C. P. J. *Carbohydr. Res.* ms. submitted.
66. Brimacombe, J. S.; Foster, A. B.; Hems, R.; Westwood, J. H.; Hall, L. D. *Can. J. Chem.* 1970, **48**, 3946.
67. Bhattacharjee, A. K.; Zissis, E.; Glaudemans, C. P.J. *Carbohydr. Res.* 1981, **89**, 249.
68. Kováč, P.; Yeh, H. C. J.; Glaudemans, C. P. J. *Carbohydr. Res.* 1985, **140**, 277.
69. Kováč, P.; Glaudemans, C. P. J. *Carbohydr. Res.* 1985, **140**, 289.
70. Kováč, P.; Glaudemans, C. P. J. *Carbohydr. Res.* 1985, **140**, 313.
71. Kováč, P.; Glaudemans, C. P. J.; Guo, W.; Wong, T. *Carbohydr. Res.* 1985, **140**, 294.
72. Gross, H.; Farkas, I.; Bognár, R. *Z. Chem.* 1978, **18**, 201.
73. Szabó, P.; Szabó, L. *J. Chem. Soc.* 1960, 3762.
74. Kováč, P. *Carbohydr. Res.* 1986, **153**, 237.

RECEIVED March 14, 1988

Chapter 7

Metabolic and Enzymatic Studies with Deoxyfluoro Carbohydrates

N. F. Taylor, D. Sbrissa, S. T. Squire[1], T. D'Amore[2], and J. M. McIntosh

Department of Chemistry and Biochemistry, University of Windsor, Windsor, Ontario N9B 3P4, Canada

The biochemical rationale for the introduction of fluorine into carbohydrates is presented and exemplified by a review of transport, metabolic and enzymatic studies with deoxyfluorosugars. Recent biochemical results with 3-deoxy-3-fluoro-D-glucose (3FG) and 4-deoxy-4-fluoro-D-glucose (4FG) illustrate the reactivity of the C-F bond. Thus unlike 3FG, when 4FG is incubated with Pseudomonas putida extensive fluoride ion release occurs due to the presence of an outer membrane protein. Using D-[6-^{3}H]-4FG and D-[U-^{14}C]-4FG a de-fluorinated metabolite is isolated and identified by ^{13}C and ^{1}H NMR analysis to be 4,5-dihydroxypentanoic acid. Evidence is also presented for the incorporation of radiolabel into a peptidylglycan fraction of the cell envelope. The specificity and kinetics of pyranose-2-oxidase (E.C. 1.1.3.10) towards glucose, 4FG and 3FG is examined. Whereas 4FG is a substrate and competitive inhibitor, 3FG is not. The synthesis of 4-deoxy-4-fluoro-D-fructose via the immobilized enzyme is also reported.

The rationale for the introduction of fluorine into carbohydrates has been extensively cited (1). Initially, the idea was based on the close similarity in size and electronegativity between fluorine and a hydroxyl group when attached to carbon (2). Support for this contention was provided by a comparative X-ray crystallographic

[1]Current address: Laboratory of Intermediary Metabolism, Institut de Recherches Clinique de Montreal, Montreal, Quebec H2W 1R7, Canada
[2]Current address: Labatts Brewing Company, Ltd., 150 Simcoe Streeet, London, Ontario N6A 4M3, Canada

analysis of erythritol and 2-deoxy-2-fluoro-DL-erythritol which revealed an almost identical crystal lattice structure for the two compounds (3). These early observations suggested that fluorine might replace a hydroxyl group in carbohydrates with minimal perturbation of molecular structure and conformation, whilst still conferring subtle differences in chemical and biochemical reactivity (4). Subsequently, a physico-chemical comparison of bond length, Van der Waals radius and electronegativity revealed a close similarity between the carbon-fluorine and carbon-oxygen bond (5). An important aspect of the biochemical rationale, emphasized by Barnett (5), is in the fact that the hydroxyl group in a carbohydrate may act as a donor or acceptor of hydrogen bonding, whilst a deoxyfluoro substituent may act only as a hydrogen bond acceptor. Thus, the replacement of the hydroxyl group by fluorine may provide useful information about the direction and stereospecificty of carbohydrate binding to a variety of proteins. There are now many in vitro and in vivo biochemical studies that support this idea (e.g. enzyme specificity and mechanism, transport proteins, antibody-antigen specificity and metabolism). Furthermore, the presence of fluorine in the substrate permits a study of substrate-protein interactions by using ^{19}F nmr spectroscopy (6). These ideas and the wider interest in the biochemistry of the carbon-fluorine bond (7,8), especially with regard to mechanism of fluoroacetate poisoning (9,10) and the concept of "lethal synthesis" developed by R.A. Peters (11), undoubtedly stimulated the growth and interest in the synthesis, reactivity and biochemistry of fluorocarbohydrates.

After a brief review of fluorocarbohydrate biochemistry in the areas of transport, enzymes and metabolism, attention will be confined to our recent metabolic and enzymatic studies with 3-deoxy-3-fluoro- and 4-deoxy-4-fluoro-D-glucose.

Transport Studies

Such studies include: 3-deoxy-3-fluoro-D-glucose and glucose transport mutants in Escherichia coli (12); 2-deoxy-2-fluoro-D-glucose and the isolation, kinetics and characterization of hexose transport mutants in L6 rat myoblasts (13,14); comparative binding studies with deoxyfluoro and deoxyhexoses to determine the structural requirements and kinetics of glucose transport in the human erythrocyte (15,16), the hamster intestine (17) and rat brain synaptosomes (18); the use of 3-deoxy-3-fluoro- and 4-deoxy-4-fluoro-D-glucose in the kinetics and characterization of the D-glucose, D-gluconate and 2-oxo-D-gluconate transport carrier systems in the cytoplasmic membrane of Pseudomonas putida (19,20). Recently (21), deoxyfluoro-sucroses have been used to study the specificity of the sucrose carrier protein in plants.

Enzyme Studies

A number of enzyme specificity studies have been undertaken based on kinetic measurements. Ideally, as in the case of transport studies, the methodology is based on a comparison of the K_m and/or the competitive K_i values of the appropriate substituted deoxyfluoro and deoxy analogue with that of the natural substrate. Such a comparison of kinetic data allows assignment of the direction and stereospecificity of hydrogen bonding of the substrate at the catalytic site of the enzyme. This approach has been used to obtain information about the specificity of glycerol kinase from Candida mycoderma (22), yeast hexokinase (22), glucosephosphate isomerase (24), galactokinase (23) and UDPG-pyrophosphorylase (26). The glucansucrases of Leuconostoc mesenteroides and Streptococcus mutans utilize sucrose as a glucosyl donor for the synthesis of glycans (27); synthetic 6-deoxy-6-fluorosucrose competitively inhibits the glucansucrases of the above organisms (Eklund, S.H.; Robyt, J.F. Carbohydr. Res. in press). Glycosyl fluorides are excellent substrates for glycosidases and they have been used to ascertain whether enzyme action occurs with or without inversion of configuration at the anomeric centre of the substrates (28-30). The enzymic hydrolysis of glycosyl fluorides is not confined to glucosidases. Thus, sucrose phosphorylase will utilize α-D-glucopyranosyl fluoride as a substrate to produce glucose-1-phosphate (31). Hence, as pointed out by Barnett (5), glycosyl fluorides are potential substrates for glycosyl transferases. The enzymatic synthesis of cyclodextrins from α-D-glucosyl fluoride and cyclodextrin- α -(1-4)glucosyltransferase has been reported (32). This use of glycosyl fluorides has also been elegantly exploited in the stereoselective synthesis of oligosacchardies by Ogawa et al (33) and is dealt with elsewhere in this book.

The binding of fluorinated sugars to enzymes has been studied with the aid of ^{19}F nmr spectroscopy (6). The addition of lysozyme to methyl N-fluoroacetyl- β -D-glucosaminide results in a downfield chemical shift in the ^{19}F nmr spectrum (34); this change in chemical shift was used to determine the binding constant. The binding of the sugar with the enzyme, in the presence of Gd^{3+}, resulted in an increase in the relaxation time of the fluorine nucleus. Since the binding site of Gd^{3+} in lysozyme was known from X-ray studies, the observed increase in relaxation time could be correlated with the conformation of the enzyme-substrate complex. Even when the fluorine spectrum is complicated by extensive fluorine coupling, it may be simplified by heteronuclear spin decoupling (35). In other studies, a comparison of the inhibition constants of a number of deoxy- and deoxyfluoroglucoses with the X-ray data of the enzyme-sugar complex has been extended to a study of the active site geometries of α-glucan phosphorylase from rabbit muscle and potatoes (36). A series of deoxyfluoro-D-glucopyranosyl phosphates have also been used to probe the mechanism of glycosyltransferase (37).

Since fluorinated sugars are frequently substrates for a variety of carbohydrate enzymes, a combination of enzymatic and chemical methods may be used for the synthesis of hitherto rather inaccessible fluorinated sugar derivatives. Thus, partially purified glucose and gluconate dehydrogenases, obtained from Pseudomonas putida have been used for the synthesis of 3-deoxy-3-fluoro- and 4-deoxy-4-fluoro-D-arabino-2-hexulosonic acids from the corresponding deoxyfluoro-D-glucoses (20,38). Even when the fluoro-sugar is a poor substrate, chemoenzymatic synthesis may be applied if a coupled re-cycling of substrate or co-factor is introduced. Immobilized yeast hexokinase when coupled to pyruvate kinase, to regenerate ATP, gives good yields of the fluorinated sugar phosphate from 3-deoxy-3-fluoro-D-glucose (3FG) (39). Subsequent lead tetraacetate oxidation of this sugar phosphate gave 2-deoxy-2-fluoro-D-arabinose-5-phosphate (2FA-5-P) (Figure 1). Undoubtedly, this approach will find many applications for the synthesis of fluorinated sugars of biochemical interest. Recently, we have used pyranose-2-oxidase for the synthesis of 4-deoxy-4-fluoro-D-fructose (40) which will be discussed later.

Metabolic Studies

The first metabolic studies were undertaken with a syrupy, chromatographically pure, but ethanol-contaminated 3-deoxy-3-fluoro-D-glucose (3FG) and hence the respirometric data reported, using Saccharomyces cerevisiae, is not valid (41). Using pure crystalline 3FG, however, and the same organism it was demonstrated that the 3FG blocked the metabolism of both glucose and galactose and inhibited polysaccharide synthesis (42,43). One possible explanation for these effects was based on the fact that 3FG-1-P and 3FG-6-P are competitive inhibitors of glucose-1-phosphate uridyltransferase and phosphoglucomutase respectively (26), in a manner similar to that proposed for the effects of 2-deoxy-D-glucose in yeast cells (44). The metabolism of 3FG and 4-deoxy-4-fluoro-D-glucose (4FG) in E. coli has been reported (45,46). In both instances, it was demonstrated that the sugars were converted to the 6-phosphates by the phosphoenolpyruvate phosphotransferase system without any further apparent metabolism. In addition, both sugars are inhibitors of cells grown on glucose or lactose as a sole carbon source. In the case of the latter, this is probably due to the demonstrated uncompetitive inhibition

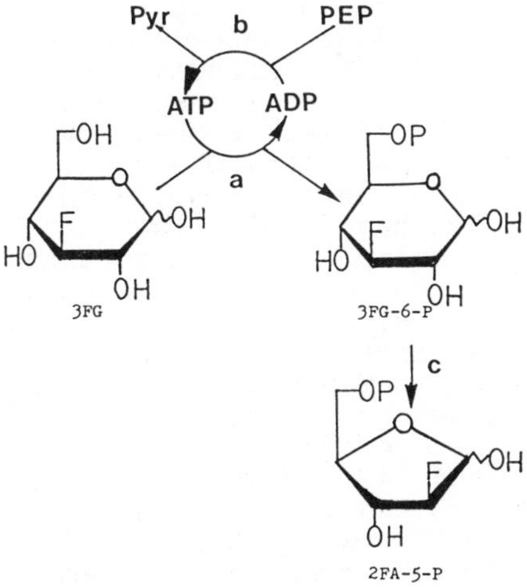

Figure 1. The chemoenzymatic synthesis of 3-deoxy-3-fluoro-D-glucose-6-phosphate (3FG-6-P) and 2-deoxy-2-fluoro-D-arabinose-5-phosphate (2FA-5-P) from 3-deoxy-3-fluoro-D-glucose (3FG). (a) Hexokinase; (b) pyruvate kinase; (c) lead tetraacetate.

of β-D-galactosidase activity by 3FG and 4FG and that 3FG-6-P and 4FG-6-P repress β-D-galactosidase synthesis. Interestingly, these results support the view that catabolite repression may be produced by compounds that are not necessarily metabolized further than the hexose-6-phosphate (47). Studies of 3FG metabolism in P. putida have also been done. Using glucose grown whole cells (48) or cell-free extracts of this organism, it was shown that 3FG is a substrate for the cytoplasmic membrane bound enzymes (49,50), glucose and gluconate dehydrogenase. The respiratory products of these two enzymes were shown to be 3-deoxy-3-fluoro-D-gluconate (3FGA) and 3-deoxy-3-fluoro-2-keto-D-gluconate (3F2KGA) respectively (51). Both 3FGA and 3F2KGA did not appear to be phosphorylated to any great extent but were competitive inhibitors of the cytosolic gluconokinase. There was no evidence of further metabolism of these fluorinated sugars via the Entner-Doudoroff pathway (52). The metabolism of the isomeric 4FG gave quite different results. Thus, unlike 3FG, no respiration could be detected with glucose grown whole cells; instead extensive fluoride ion was detected in the cell supernatants. With cell free extracts of this organism, however, no fluoride ion was detected and the correct stoichiometric respiration of the 4FG was observed for the formation of 4-deoxy-4-fluoro-D-gluconate (4FGA) and 4-deoxy-4-fluoro-2-keto-D-gluconate (4F2KGA). Further studies indicated that the de-fluorination of 4FG was due to the presence of an inducible/repressible protein located in the outer membrane of the cell envelope (53). More recent aspects of this metabolism will be discussed later.

A number of studies on the metabolism of 3FG and 4FG in Locusta migratoria have been undertaken. Both 3FG and 4FG are toxic to locust with LD50's of 4.8 mg/g and 0.6 mg/g respectively. In vitro studies showed that 3FG is metabolized in the fat body, via the NADP-linked aldose reductase, to 3-deoxy-3-fluoro-D-glucitol (3FGL). This metabolite was detected in the hemolymph of the insect and shown to be both a competitive inhibitor and a substrate for NAD-linked sorbitol dehydrogenase, thereby generating 3-deoxy-3-fluoro-D-fructose (3FF) (54). Subsequently, it was shown by in vivo radio-respirometric analysis of $^{14}CO_2$ and appropriate chase experiments, that 3FG metabolism irreversibly inhibits glycolysis and not the hexose monophosphate shunt or tricarboxylic acid cycle (55). In addition, the release of fluoride ion and ^3H_2O from D-[3-^{3}H]-3FG was also observed. Based on the mechanism of aldolase (56) and triosephosphate isomerase (57), 3FG is probably metabolized as far as pro-R-^{3}H-monofluorohydroxyacetone phosphate and glyceraldehyde-3-phosphate (GA-3-P) (Figure 2). It has been demonstrated with fat body and flight muscle extracts that, in addition to the above events, D-[3-^{3}H]-3FG is incorporated into tritium-labeled glycogen and trehalose

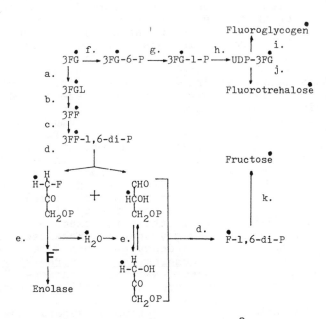

Figure 2. Proposed metabolism of D-(3-^{3}H)-3FG in
Locusta migratoria. ●Tritium label. 3FG, 3-deoxy-3-
fluoro-D-glucose; 3FGL, 3-deoxy-3-fluoro-D-glucitol;
3FF, 3-deoxy-3-fluoro-D-fructose; UDP, uridine
diphosphate. Enzymes: (a) aldose reductase; (b)
sorbitol dehydrogenase; (c) fructokinases; (d)
aldolase; (e) triosephosphate isomerase; (f) hexokinase; (g) phosphoglucomutase; (h) UDP-glucose pyrophosphorylase; (i) glycogen synthetase; (j) trehalose
synthetase; (k) fructose phosphatases. Fluoride ion
and tritiated water have been measured; tritium labeled
fluoroglycogen, fluorotrehalose, 3FGL and fructose
have been identified.

(58) (Figure 2). The formation of "fluoroglycogen" and "fluorotrehalose" was confirmed by Fourier transform ^{19}F NMR analysis of the chromatographically separated fractions. The inhibition of trehalase by "fluorotrehalose" was also suggested by the accumulation of radiolabeled trehalose. Inhibition of trehalase by 6-deoxy-6-fluorotrehalose has been reported (59). In addition, there is an accumulation of tritium labeled fructose. This result is consistent with the observed release of ^3H_2O and fluoride ion from pro-R-^{3}H-mono-fluorohydroxyacetone phosphate, which in the presence of triosephosphate isomerase, would equilibrate with the formation of ^{3}H-dihydroxyacetone phosphate and ^{3}H-GA-3-P. The inhibition of enolase by fluoride ion (60) and the action of aldolase would allow the accumulation of the tritium labeled fructose (Figure 2). These studies illustrate how a fluorinated sugar may utilize a number of catabolic and anabolic enzymes, involving both retention and cleavage of the C-F bond, to exert a novel type of "Lethal Synthesis". The structural elucidation of "fluoroglycogen" and "fluorotrehalose" remain to be established as well as the specificity of the enzymes involved. Although this is the first example of fluoro sugar incorporation into glycogen or trehalose, it has been reported that 4-deoxy-4-fluoro-D-mannose is metabolized in Saccharomyces cerevisiae to guanosinediphosphate-4-deoxy-4-fluoro-D-mannose, with possible incorporation into cell wall polysaccharide (61).

The metabolism of deoxyfluoro sugars has been studied in relation to the inhibition of glycoprotein biosynthesis. Thus, 2-deoxy-2-fluoro-D-glucose (2FG) and 2-deoxy-2-fluoro-D-mannose (2FM) are potent inhibitors of enveloped virus multiplication. The inhibition is considered to be due to the metabolism of the fluorinated sugars to the guanosinediphosphate (GDP) and uridinediphosphate (UDP) derivatives. The inhibition of viral multiplication and glycoprotein biosynthesis is relieved by the addition of glucose or mannose, the latter being more effective. Both GDP-2-deoxy-2-fluoro-D-glucose (GDP2FG) and GDP-2-deoxy-2-fluoro-D-mannose (GDP2FM) compete, therefore, with GDP-mannose as inhibitors of protein glycosylation (62,63). It has been shown that the enzyme that transfers oligosaccharides from lipid carrier to protein recognizes the complete fully glycosylated oligosaccharide (64). Since GDP2FG and GDP2FM prevent the completion of the lipid-linked oligosaccharides, intermediate oligosaccharide fragments can be isolated from such cells. The formation of smaller oligosaccharides is prevented by the addition of mannose and glycosylation of the protein is restored (65). More detailed in vivo and in vitro studies on 2FG inhibition of protein glycosylation in influenza A virus infected chick embryo cells have been reported (66,67). In recent studies, using chemically synthesized UDP2FG and GDP2FM, it has been shown that the latter compound in a cell-free system, inhibits the synthesis of Man-(GlcNAc)$_2$-PP-dolichol from (GlcNAc)$_2$-PP-dolichol and GDP-man (68). Thus further assembly of the tetradecasaccharide precursor, Glc$_3$-Man$_9$-(GlcNAc)$_2$-PP-dolichol carrier (69), which is required for protein glycosylation, is prevented. The metabolism of 4-deoxy-4-fluoro-D-mannose (4FM) and 4-deoxy-D-mannose (4dM) has also been examined. Both analogues have been shown to be metabolized in yeast to their respective 6-phosphates (70) and they interfere with the glycosylation of viral G-protein in VSV (vesicular stomatitis virus) infected BHK (British Hamster Kidney) cells (71). In order to investigate these inhibitory effects, GDP4FM and GDP4dM have been synthesized and their effects on the dolichol pathway in vitro in chick embryo cell microsomal membranes and in vivo in BHK cells have been examined (McDowell, W.; Grier, T.J.; Rasmussen, J.R.; Schwarz, R.T. Biochem. J., in press). In the microsomal studies, GDP4FM blocked the addition of mannose to Man-(GlcNAc)$_2$-PP-Dolichol and was a very poor substrate for GDP-Man:Dol-P-mannosyl transferase. Dol-P-4FM could only be synthesized in vitro if chick embryo cell membranes were primed with Dol-P. Thus, the observed inhibition of lipid-linked oligosaccharide formation in BHK cells, treated with 4FM, is considered to be due primarily to a blockage in the formation of Man$_2$-(GlcNAc)$_2$-PP-Dolichol by GDP4FM. In contrast, GDP4dM was a substrate for the Dol-P-mannosyl transferase and in BHK cells, Man$_9$-(GlcNAc)$_2$-PP-Dolichol was the major lipid linked oligosaccharide detected; almost normal levels of protein glycosylation were observed. The formation of more complex oligosaccharides was inhibited and the high mannose structures detected were smaller than in the case of untreated cells. Recently, in a kinetic study,(McDowell, Justus Liebig Universitat, Giessen, personal communication, 1987) has measured the inhibition constants (Ki values) of a number of GDP-mannose analogues for GDP-Man:Dol-P-mannosyl transferase in chick embryo cell microsomes. It was found the GDP4dM > GDP-3-deoxymannose > GDP-4-deoxymannose > GDP-2-deoxymannose >>> GDP4FM. All the nucleoside diphosphate analogues, with the exception of GDP-4-deoxy-4-fluoromannose, readily formed Dolichol-P-sugar derivatives. As previously observed, Dol-P-4FM is only formed if the microsomes are primed with Dol-P. From these results, the specificity of the enzyme for position C4 of mannose would appear to be critical. Thus, the replacement of the C4 hydroxyl group in mannose by fluorine may change the direction of hydrogen bonding normally required for enzyme substrate binding.

Finally, an important area of medical research which is beyond the scope of this review, involves the use of ^{18}F fluorinated carbohydrates in the Positron Emission

Transaxial Tomography (PETT) technique. This technology
permits the use of fluorinated sugars as non-invasive
probes of metabolic flux in animals and humans (72,73).
[2-^{18}F]-2-deoxy-2-fluoro-D-glucose [2-^{18}FG] and [3-^{18}F]-
3-deoxy-3-fluoro-D-glucose [3-^{18}FG] have been used to
study the regional cerebral metabolic rate (rCMR) for
glucose. These sugars are trapped in the brain tissue,
after rate limiting phosphorylation by hexokinase, and
permit, therefore, PETT scans 30-40 minutes after
administration of the labeled sugar (73). Using 2-^{18}FG,
the effects of different sensory stimuli on the rCMR have
been used to obtain the metabolic mapping of functional
activity in the brain (74). The regional variations in
rCMR in a variety of pathological conditions of the
brain such as convulsive disorders, Huntington's chorea,
neoplastic conditions and schizophrenia have been
explored by the same technique (75).

Further Studies with 4-Deoxy-4-fluoro-D-glucose and P. Putida

As discussed earlier, 3FG is oxidized by P. putida
(Scheme 1a). 4-Deoxy-4-fluoro-D-glucose (4FG), however,
is metabolized, in glucose grown cells of P. putida,
without respiration but with extensive (> 95%) fluoride
ion release (Scheme 1b). Fractionation of the cell
envelope (76) indicated that this C-F bond cleavage in
4FG is confined to a peptidylglycan associated protein of
the organism. No C-F bond cleavage is observed with cell-
free extracts or the cytoplasmic membrane fraction.
Instead, 4FG is oxidized, to the extent of 2 g atoms of
oxygen/mol, by the cytoplasmic membrane bound enzymes
glucose oxidase (GOX) and gluconate dehydrogenase (GDH)
(49,50). The products of oxidation are 4-deoxy-4-fluoro-
D-gluconate (4FGA) and 2-keto-4-deoxy-4-fluoro-D-
gluconate (2K4FGA) respectively (Scheme 1c).

Scheme 1

(a) whole cells: 3FG $\xrightarrow{\text{GOX}}$ 3FGA $\xrightarrow{\text{GDH}}$ 2K3FGA

(b) whole cells: 4FG $\longrightarrow$ F$^-$ + defluorinated product(s)

(c) cell-free extracts: 4FG $\xrightarrow{\text{GOX}}$ 4FGA $\xrightarrow{\text{GDH}}$ 2K4FGA

Using chloroamphenicol treated glucose or succinate grown
cells, it was also demonstrated that the defluorination
was due to the presence of an inducible/respressible
protein. The fluoride release from 4FG by
chloroamphenicol treated glucose grown cells, displayed
saturation kinetics (Km, 3.6 m; Vmax, 1 nmol fluoride/mg
protein/min) and could be prevented in the presence of
glucose, gluconate and 2-ketogluconate. Further, the
complete protection of fluoride release was achieved in

the   presence   of   N-ethyl   maleimide   which   suggested   the
involvement   of   a   protein -SH group   in   the   C-F   bond
cleavage.   These results are considered to be   consistent
with   an initial equilibrium binding of 4FG (by   possible
fluorine-hydrogen bonding) to an -SH containing   protein,
followed by a slow fluoride elimination or displacement.
    In order to investigate the pathway and mechanism of
fluoride   release   from   4FG   further,   we   initially
synthesized   4-deoxy-4-fluoro-D-[6-^{3}H]glucose   (D-[6-^{3}H]-
4FG) (77). Incubation of glucose grown whole cells of P.
putida   with the radiolabeled 4FG (specific activity   7.2
mCi/mmol),   however, gave an unexpected result. Thus, a 24
h incubation of the organism with 1 mM D-[6-^{3}H]-4FG   gave
100% fluoride release as well as an unexpected   extensive
release   of   radiolabel   from   the   substrate.   After
centrifugation,   approximately   70%   of   the   total
radioactivity was found in the supernatant fraction, with
the remainder in the cell pellet. Approximately 1% of the
radioactivity   remained   cell   envelope   associated   after
extensive   dialysis   of   the   cell   pellet.   Borate   anion-
exchange column analysis (78) of the supernatant fraction
demonstrated   that the loss of radioactivity was   due   to
^{3}H$_2$O   (Figure   3, Peak A) and that a   significant   amount
(20%)   of a tritiated unidentified component (Figure   3,
Peak   B)   was   produced. Peak   B   was   shown,   by
chromatographic   and Fourier transform ^{19}F NMR   analysis,
to be a non-fluorinated acidic carbohydrate.
    To   overcome the extensive tritium loss   encountered
with   D-[6-^{3}H]-4FG,   we have now   synthesized   4-deoxy-4-
fluoro-D-[U-^{14}C]-glucose (D-[U-^{14}C]-4FG) by the action of
diethylaminosulphur   trifluoride on   methyl   2,3,6-tri-O-
benzoyl- α -D-[U-^{14}C]galactopyranoside   (Sbrissa   and
Taylor,   unpublished   results). Table   I   summarizes   the
distribution   of   radioactivity   in   various   fractions
obtained   from a 24 h incubation of glucose   grown   whole
cells of P. putida (600 mg protein) with 1 mM   D-[U-^{14}C]-
4FG   (specific   activity: 10,600 dpm/umol)   in 0.1   M,   pH
7.1,   potassium phosphate buffer, at 30°C.   Fluoride   ion
measurements   in the supernatant fractions indicated a   95
± 5% release of F$^-$ in two incubations. Additionally,   two
independent   smaller scale incubations, designed to   trap
any liberated carbon dioxide, showed that as much as   4.8
± 0.2% of the radiolabel was lost as ^{14}CO$_2$. When   the
supernatant   fraction, which accounted for more than   50%
of the initial radioactivity (Table I), was submitted   to
borate   anion-exchange column chromatography   and   eluted
with   a   linear   ammonium   tetraborate   gradient,   the
radiolabeled   material was resolved into a single   poorly
retained   "minor   peak" and a   strongly   retained   "major
peak"   metabolite. Internal carbohydrate standards   were
detected at 420 nm by the orcinol colourimetric procedure
(79),   (Figure   4).   A   similar   control   chromatographic
analysis   of a sample obtained from a 24 h incubation   of
1.0   mM D-[U-^{14}C]-4FG under identical conditions, in   the

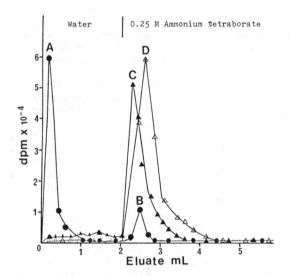

Figure 3. Dowex AB 1-X8 borate resin micro-column estimation of tritiated water released from 1 mM D-(6-^{3}H)-4FG after 24 h incubation with P. putida. Column applications: ● 25 μL cell supernatant; peak A, tritiated water, eluted with water; peak B, unidentified defluorinated carbohydrate; ▲ 25 μL of 1 mM D-(6-^{3}H)-4FG, peak C; △ 25 μL 1 mM D-(U-^{14}C)-glucose, peak D. All carbohydrates were eluted with 0.25 M ammonium tetraborate.

absence of cells, gave less than 1% release of F⁻ and
unchanged 4FG. Isolation of the major-peak metabolite by
preparative borate column chromatography and thin layer
chromatographic analysis, yielded a single radiolabeled
product. The 75 MHz proton-coupled (Figure 5), proton-
decoupled ^{13}C NMR (Figure 6) of this product indicated
the presence of one -CH, three CH_2 groups and one
carbonyl group. Four absorptions were present in the 300
MHz proton NMR (Figure 7). The chemical shift of two of
these, 3.67 (1H) and 3.53 (2H), correspond to protons on
oxygenated carbon (M and L respectively) and another,
2.27 (2H), corresponded to protons adjacent to a carbonyl
group. No methyl groups were evident ensuring that the
chain was terminated by an oxygenated carbon. 2D proton
NMR (COSY-90 pulse sequence) allowed a complete
determination of the structure. Cross peaks indicating
coupling appeared only between protons K and J, J and M
and M and L. The structure 4,5-dihydroxypentanoic acid
(2,3-dideoxy-D-ribonic acid), (1) in Figure 7, is the
only one which will accommodate these data.

Table I.   Distribution of radioactivity in P. putida
            after 24 h incubation with 1 mM D-[U-^{14}C]4FG

Fraction	Radioactivity* (dpm)	% of Initial radioactivity
Supernatant	555,955	52.4
Whole Cell dialysate	368,625	34.8
Supernatant from dialysis bag	8,177	0.8
Cell envelope	4,497	0.42
Cell-free extract (after dialysis)	54,779	5.2
Trapped CO_2 (from whole cells)	50,858	4.8
Residual material	15,785	1.5
Recovery		99.2

* Based on two identical incubations.

The stereochemistry at C4 is probably D although this has
yet to be unequivocally established. The structure of (1)
was further supported by a FAB mass spectrum which
yielded a single intense peak with a m/e ratio of 133,
corresponding to the expected molecular weight of the
carboxylate anion. A final confirmation of the structure
was obtained when the ^{13}C proton-decoupled NMR of (1)
(Figure 6) was shown to be identical to authentic DL-4,5-
dihydroxypentanoic acid (**80**).
    An investigation of the non-dialysable radiolabel
incorporated into the cell envelope fraction (Table 1)
was now undertaken. A sodium dodecylsulphate (SDS)
solubilized sample of this fraction was submitted to gel

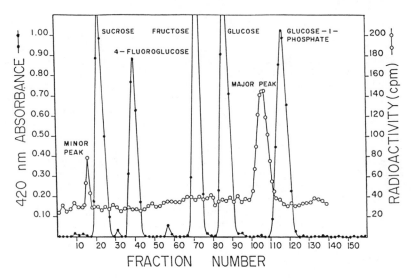

Figure 4. Dowex-1-X8 borate anion-exchange column chromatographic analysis of supernatants from 24 hour incubations of
P. putida with 4-deoxy-4-fluoro-D-(U-^{14}C)glucose. O Radiolabeled
metabolites; ● internal non-radiolabeled carbohydrate standards.
All compounds were eluted with a linear gradient of ammonium
tetraborate.

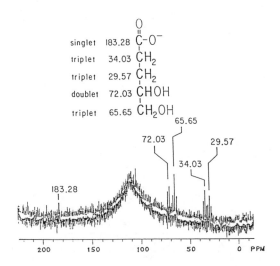

Figure 5. Proton-coupled ^{13}C NMR spectrum of the major metabolite
isolated from P. putida after a 24 hour incubation with 4-deoxy-
4-fluoro-D-(U-^{14}C)glucose. The carbon-13 Fourier transformed
NMR spectrum was obtained with a 300 MHz General Electric NMR
spectrometer after 36000 scans in D_2O. Chemical shift values
(PPM) are relative to tetramethylsilane.

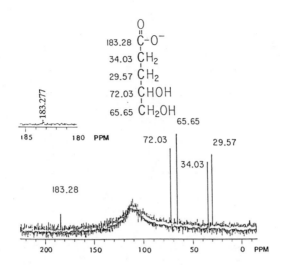

Figure 6. Proton-decoupled ^{13}C NMR spectrum of the major metabolite isolated from P. putida after 24 hour incubation with 4-deoxy-4-fluoro-D-(U-^{14}C)glucose. Conditions the same as in Figure 5.

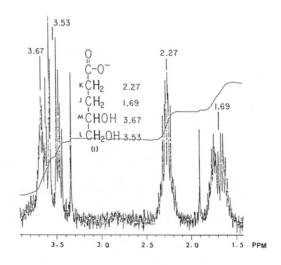

Figure 7. Proton Fourier transformed NMR spectrum of the major metabolite isolated from P. putida after 24 hour incubation with 4-deoxy-4-fluoro-D-(U-^{14}C)glucose. The spectrum was obtained after 8 scans using the same conditions as in Figure 5.

filtration on a BioGel A-1.5m column. As can be seen (Figure 8), all the radiolabel is covalently associated with a component (Peak A) of molecular weight > 400,000 which corresponds to the void volume (Vo). Treatment of the same cell envelope fraction with lysozyme, prior to solubilization with SDS and identical gel filtration, revealed that the radiolabeled material has now migrated to a component (Figure 9, Peak B) with a molecular weight < 14,000. These results indicate a covalent attachment of radiolabel to a peptidylglycan present in the cell envelope which is degraded to smaller fragments by lysozyme. The chemical nature of this incorporation into the cell wall and the biochemical events leading to it, remains to be established.

A hypothetical pathway for the loss of ^3H_2O from D-[6-^{3}H]-4FG is proposed in Figure 10. The kinetic data support an equilibrium binding of 4FG (2) to an outer membrane protein (3), followed by an irreversible loss of F^- at C4 and a proton at C5 to form the hexoseen (4). The acyclic form (5) of (4) may now rearrange by prototropy to give the equilibrated forms: (5) $\rightleftharpoons$ (6) $\rightleftharpoons$ (7). This would be consistent with the observed exchange of tritium at C6 with water (Figure 3). The precise metabolic pathway for the formation of 2,3-dideoxy-D-ribonic acid (1) remains to be established. The observed production of $^{14}CO_2$ (Table I) by an oxidative-decarboxylation of a non-fluorinated metabolite of D-[U-^{14}C]-4FG, however, does account for the isolation of the 5-carbon sugar (1).

The Specificity of Pyranose-2-oxidase and the Synthesis of 4-Deoxy-4-fluoro-D-fluoro-D-fructose

Pyranose-2-oxidase (E.C. 1.1.3.10), isolated from the mycelia of Polyporus obtusus, has been reported to oxidize-D-glucose and other carbohydrates at C2 to yield the 2-keto derivatives (81-85). The enzyme which exists as a single protein band on acrylamide gel, is a tetramer consisting of identical subunits, each of a molecular weight of 68,000 and a total molecular weight of 220,000 (86). Janssen and Ruelius (81) showed that modification of the β-D-gluco configuration at C2, C3 or C4, led to more than a 90% decrease in enzyme activity. Since no kinetic details for this enzyme and its substrates were available, especially with regard to fluorocarbohydrates, a kinetic analysis has been undertaken.

A Lineweaver-Burk plot (87) indicates that with D-glucose as the substrate, the enzyme obeys Michaelis-Menten kinetics with a Km value of 3.2 ± 0.08 mM and a Vmax of 126.0 ± 0.02 micromol/mg protein/min (Figure 11). Similar results were obtained by the direct linear plot (88), Hanes and Woolf (89) or Eadie-Hofstee plots (90). All the kinetic data reported here and subsequently, were based on the initial rates of hydrogen peroxide formation

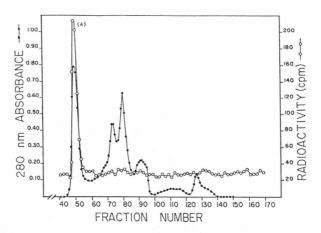

Figure 8. BioGel A 1.5m column chromatographic analysis of SDS-solubilized cell envelope isolated from P. putida after 24 hour incubation with 4-deoxy-4-fluoro-D-(U-C^{14})glucose. O Radiolabeled fraction; ● cell envelope proteins.

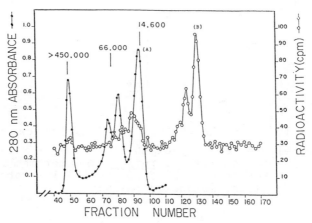

Figure 9. BioGel A 1.5m column chromatographic analysis of the cell envelope isolated from P. putida after 24 hour incubation with 4-deoxy-4-fluoro-D-(U-^{14})glucose and treatment with lysozyme. O Radiolabeled lysozyme treated cell envelope fraction, peak B;●cell envelope proteins plus lysozyme, peak A. The vertical bars correspond to the molecular weight range.

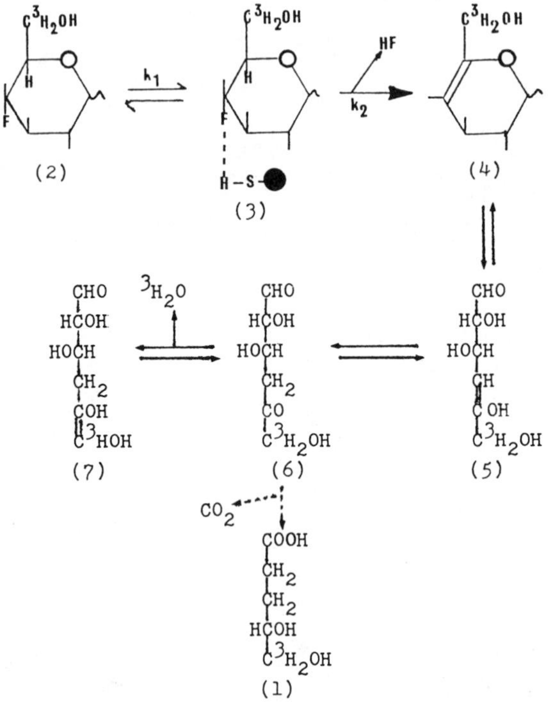

Figure 10. Possible pathway for fluoride and tritiated water release from 4-deoxy-4-fluoro-D-(6-^{3}H)glucose after incubation with P. putida. ● Outer membrane protein. The conversion of (6) to (1) is probably by an intracellular metabolic pathway.

from the enzyme and substrate (81). 4FG was also a comparatively good substrate with a Km value of 5.54 ± 0.64 mM and a Vmax of 104.0 ± 0.07 micromol/mg protein/min (Figure 11).

As expected 4FG was a competitive inhibitor of glucose with a Ki value of 5.50 ± 0.02 mM (Figure 12). Glucose, however, was a poorer competitive inhibitor when 4FG was the substrate with a Ki value of 24.90 ± 0.25 mM (data not shown). Presumably, due to the hydrogen bonding capacity of fluorine at C4, 4FG binds more effectively as an enzyme-substrate complex. As with 3-O-methyl-D-glucose (81), the C3 modified fluoro-analogue, 3FG was not a substrate for the enzyme. It was of interest to observe, however, that the Vmax of glucose was substantially increased in the presence of increasing concentrations of 3FG (Figure 13). This kinetic pattern is similar to that observed by Krupka (91) with acetylcholine esterase and a number of choline analogues. The result was explained by the interaction of the anionic component of the analogue with a positively charged site, some distance from the catalytic site of the enzyme. A similar interaction between the electronegative fluorine atom in 3FG and a cationic site of pyranose-2-oxidase may occur. Alternatively, 3FG may react with the enzyme and release fluoride ion which then allosterically enhances the enzyme activity. Preliminary experiments support this latter hypothesis. Thus, when 5.0 mL of 16 mM 3FG was reacted with the pyranose-2-oxidase (79 microg protein), a 95% fluoride ion release was detected. Further studies are required to elucidate the kinetics and mechanism of this 3FG interaction with the enzyme. It is of interest to note, that in a previous report (92) fluoride ion was found to stimulate the accumulation of D-arabino-hexo-2-ulose during the oxidation of glucose by pyranose-2-oxidase.

The chemical synthesis of deoxyfluoro-D-fructoses has been restricted to 1-deoxy-1-fluoro-D-fructose (93) and 1,6-dideoxy-1,6-difluoro-D-fructose (94). The introduction of fluorine into other positions of this sugar continues to pose a challenge (95,96). A successful chemoenzymatic synthesis of D-fructose from D-glucose, and the immobilized pyranose-2-oxidase, however, has been reported (97). Since 4FG is a substrate for this enzyme, an identical synthesis of 4-deoxy-4-fluoro-D-fructose (9) was undertaken (Figure 14). Incubation of 4FG with the immobilized enzyme on Sepharose 4B for 28 h and HPLC analysis (BioRadAminex HPX 87 H column), led to the disappearance of 4FG and the appearance of a product with a slower retention time. This product was isolated as a syrup which failed to crystallize. IR analysis indicated the presence of a new strong carbonyl stretching vibration at 1690 cm^{-1} and the presence of the C-F bond at 1350 cm^{-1} which was consistent with the structure of 4-deoxy-4-fluoro-D-arabino-hexos-2-ulose (8) (Figure 14).

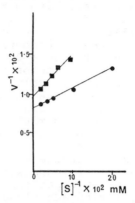

Figure 11. Pyranose-2-oxidase; Lineweaver-Burk plots.
● Glucose; Km, 3.2 mM; Vmax, 126 micromol/min/mg
protein. ■ 4-Deoxy-4-fluoro-D-glucose; Km, 5.5 mM;
Vmax, 104 micromol/min/mg protein. Each point
represents the mean of three determinations. Data
plotted by the method of least squares. S, substrate
concentration (mM); V, micromol hydrogen peroxide/
min/mg protein.

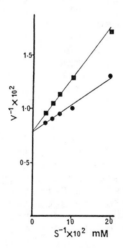

Figure 12. Pyranose-2-oxidase. Competitive inhibition
of glucose oxidation by 4-deoxy-4-fluoro-D-glucose.
● Glucose; ■ glucose in the presence of 15 mM
inhibitor. Data obtained as in Figure 11. V, micro-
mol/min/mg protein; S, glucose concentration (mM).

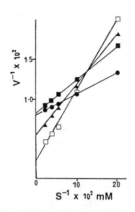

Figure 13. Pyranose-2-oxidase. The effect of increasing concentrations of 3-deoxy-3-fluoro-D-glucose on the activity of the enzyme toward glucose. ● glucose only; in the presence of: ■ 5 mM, ▲ 10 mM, □ 15 mM 3-deoxy-3-fluoro-D-glucose. Data obtained as in Figure 11. V, micromol/min/mg protein; S, glucose conentration (mM).

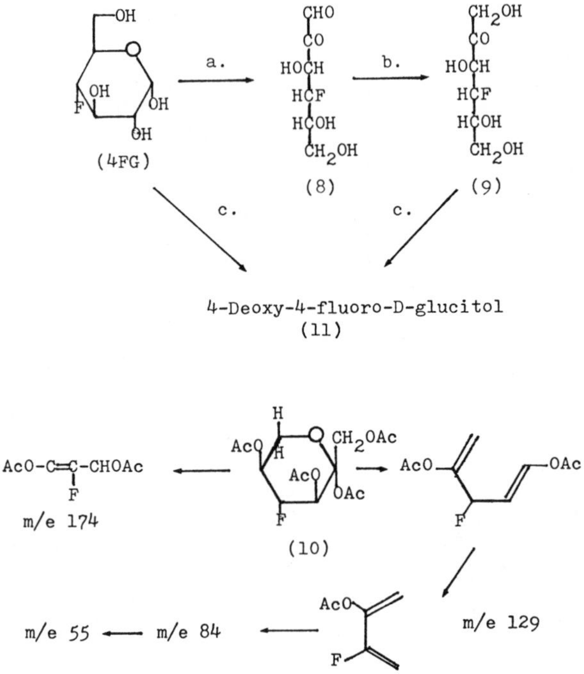

Figure 14.   The chemoenzymatic synthesis of 4-deoxy-4-fluoro-
D-fructose and some mass spectrum peaks of the peracetylated
derivative.   (a) Immobilized pyranose-2-oxidase; (c) sodium
borohydride reduction.   The observed m/e 129, derived from
(10), is diagnostic for a 2-ketopyranose.

The structure of this compound was supported by a comparative electron impact mass spectrometric analysis of the derivatized glucose, glucosone and 4-deoxy-4-fluoroglucosone (8) (Table II). All the sugars were rendered volatile by conversion to the peracetylated hydrazones or osazones by established procedures (96). The tri-O-acetyl-diphenylhydrazone of (8) showed intense mass ion peaks at m/e 472 (M^+,$C_{24}H_{25}N_2O_7F$) and 223 ($C_{14}H_{11}H_2O$: O-C-C-H=N-N(Ph)$_2$), whilst the corresponding glucosone showed peaks at 512 (M^+, $C_{26}H_{28}N_2O_9$) and 223. The common peaks at 223 are diagnostic for the glucosone structure (92,97). The 40 mass unit difference between peaks 472 and 512, derived from the hydrazones of (8) and glucosone, is due to the presence of fluorine (m/e, 19) instead of acetoxy (m/e, 59) respectively (Table II). Similarly, the mass unit differences with corresponding osazones were found to be consistent with their respective structures.

After isolation, (8) was subjected to catalytic hydrogenation (Pd/C). HPLC analysis of the reaction mixture showed the formation of a new component (9) isolated as a syrup which failed to crystallize. Although not crystalline, the tetra-O-acetyl derivatives of (9) gave the correct elemental analysis and mass spectrometric fragmentation pattern for the formation of 4-deoxy-4-fluoro-tetra-O-acetyl- αβ -D-fructopyranose (10) (α-isomer shown Figure 14). This is based on the fragmentation of peracetylated fluoro-hexoses and pentoses previously discussed (98).

Table II. Comparison of major mass spectrum peaks from diphenylhydrazone O-acetylated derivatives of glucose (a), glucosone (b) and 4-deoxy-4-fluoro-glucosone (c)

Diphenylhydrazones			
(a) Penta-O- acetate m/e	(b) Tetra-O- acetate m/e	(c) Tri-O- acetate m/e	Fragment
556	512	472	Hydrazone (mol.ion)
	223	223	OC-CH=NN(Ph)$_2$ diagnostic for glucosone
145	145	145	CH$_3$CO-O-COCH$_3$ (with H above O)
103	103	103	CH$_3$CO-O-COCH$_3$ (with OCCH$_3$ above)
43	43	43	CH$_3$CO$^+$

Thus (10) will differ from 4FG by an interchange of substituents at C1 and C5. As a result, the peracetylated pyranose form of (9) will be more highly substituted at the ketal carbon than the corresponding form of 4FG. Consequently, as observed (Figure 14), (10) will be split at C6 and C3 leading to m/e fragments 129, 84 and 55. The presence of the fluorine in (10) at C4 also makes the cleavage between C4-C5 and C4-C3 unfavourable (98) resulting, in this case, with a mass unit of 174. The structure of 4-deoxy-4-fluoro-D-fructose (9) was further confirmed by sodium borohydride reduction to an alditol which was shown to be identical (optical rotation, IR and ^{19}F NMR) to 4-deoxy-4-fluoro-D-glucitol (11), obtained by a similar reduction of 4FG.

Conclusion and Future Perspectives

Our studies with ^{14}C and tritiated 4-deoxy-4-fluoro-D-glucose (4FG) demonstrate that this sugar is metabolized in whole cells of P. putida with cleavage of the C-F bond. The isomeric 3-deoxy-3-fluoro-D-glucose (3FG), however, is metabolized with retention of the C-F bond. This stereospecific defluorination of 4FG appears to be initiated by an inducible/repressible protein associated with the outer membrane which is involved with the uptake of glucose, gluconate and 2-ketogluconate. Subsequent intracellular metabolism of the defluorinated sugar, via decarboxylation of an as yet unknown metabolite, leads to the formation of a 5-carbon sugar, identified as 2,3-dideoxyribonic acid. In addition to the above events, a significant amount of radiolabel is incorporated into the peptidylglycan component of the cell wall. The C-F bond is considered to be the strongest single bond (450-485 kJ) formed by carbon (99). Clearly, in a biological milieu, this situation is not applicable. This is further illustrated with the enzyme pyranose-2-oxidase, isolated from Polyporus obtusus. Thus, 4FG is a substrate whereas interaction of the enzyme with the isomeric 3FG results in C-F bond cleavage and fluoride ion is released. The mechanism of this defluorination and the apparent allosteric stimulation of the catalytic activity of the enzyme, remains to be determined.

Immediate future studies with P. putida are: the isolation and function of the outer membrane protein and to establish the mechanism of fluoride release from 4FG; elucidate the pathway intermediates for the metabolism of 4FG to 2,3-dideoxyribonic acid in whole cells by high resolution wide bore NMR spectrometry (100); ascertain the location and nature of the radiolabel incorporated into the peptidylglycan component. Whether the incorporation leads to a modified peptidylglycan (cell wall) is a question of particular interest in relation to the effects on cell growth. Preliminary experiments show that 4FG inhibits the growth of P. putida and P.

aeruginosa. In the longer term, whether this form of 4FG metabolism is confined to the Pseudomonads or is applicable to other gram-negative bacteria, remains to be determined.

In general, when the C-F bond is retained, the early biochemical rationale for the synthesis of deoxyfluorinated sugars has now been illustrated by numerous examples. Our own studies indicate that deoxyfluoro sugars may serve as novel membrane, enzyme and metabolic probes. Additionally, as a result of demonstrated incorporation and/or "lethal synthesis", fluorinated sugars have considerable potential to augment the antibiotic and antiviral arsenal.

Acknowledgments

One of us (NFT) thanks the Natural Sciences and Engineering Research Council, Canada (NSERC), for continued support, without which much of this work would not have been possible. The awards of an NSERC Scholarship (TD), an Ontario Graduate Scholarship (DS) and a University of Windsor Scholarship (STS) are gratefully acknowledged.

Literature Cited

1. Penglis, A.A.E. Adv. Carbohydr. Chem. Biochem. 1981, 38, 195-285.
2. Taylor, N.F.; Kent, P.W. J. Chem. Soc. 1958, 168, 872-875.
3. Bekoe, A.; Powell, H.M. Proc. R. Soc. Ser. A. 1959, 250, 301-315.
4. Kent, P.W. Chem. Ind. (London) 1969, 1128-1132.
5. Barnett, J.E.G. In Ciba Fdn. Symp. Carbon Fluorine Compounds; Elsevier & Associated Scientific Publishers, Amsterdam, 1972; 95-115.
6. Dwek, R.A. In Ciba Fdn. Symp. Carbon Fluorine Compounds; Elsevier & Associated Scientific Publishers, Amsterdam, 1972; 239-279.
7. Ciba Fdn. Symp.: Carbon-Fluorine Compounds; Elsevier & Associated Scientific Publishers, Amsterdam, 1972, 1-417.
8. Biochemistry Involving Carbon-Fluorine Bonds: Filler, R., Ed.; ACS Symposium Series 28, American Chemical Society, Washington, D.C., 1976, 1-214.
9. Peters, R.A.; Wakelin, R.W.; Buffa, P.; Thomas, L.C. Proc. R. Soc. Ser. B 1953, 140, 497-506.
10. Kirsten, E.; Sharma, M.L.; Kun, E. Molec. Pharmacol. 1978, 14, 172-184.
11. Peters, R.A. In Biochemical Lesions and Lethal Synthesis; Alexander, P. and Bacq, Z.M., Eds. Pergamon Press, Oxford, 1963, 88-130.
12. Kornberg, H.L.; Smith, J. FEBS Lett. 1972, 20 270-272.

13. D'Amore, T.; Duronio, V.; Cheung, M.O.; Lo, T.C.Y. J. Cell. Physiol. 1986, 126, 29-36.

14. D'Amore, T.; Lo, T.C.Y. J. Cell Physiol. 1986, 127, 95-105.

15. Barnett, J.E.G.; Holman, J.D.; Chalkley, R.A.; Biochem. J. 1975, Biochem. J. 145, 417-4229.

16. Lopes, D.P.; Taylor, N.F. Carbohydr. Res. 1979, 73, 124-134.

17. Barnett, J.E.G.; Holman, J.D.; Munday, K.A. Biochem. J. 1973, 131, 24-221.

18. Halton, D.M.; Taylor, N.F.; Lopes, D. J. Neurosci. Res. 1980, 5, 241-252.

19. Al-Jobore, A.; Moses, G.C.; Taylor, N.F. Can. J. Biochem. 1980, 58, 1397-1404.

20. Agbanyo, F.R.; Taylor, N.F. Biochem. J. 1983, 223, 257-262.

21. Schmalstig, J.G.; Hitz, W.D. Plant Physiol. 1987, 85, 407-12.

22. Eisenthal, R.; Harrison, R.; Lloyd, W.J.; Taylor, N.F. Biochem. J. 1972, 130, 199-205.

23. Bessell, E.M.; Foster, A.B.; Westwood, J.H. Biochem. J. 1972 128, 199-204.

24. Bessell, E.M.; Thomas, P. Biochem. J. 1972, 131, 77-82.

25. Thomas, P.; Bessell, E.M.; Westwood, J.H. Biochem. J. 1974, 139, 661-664.

26. Wright, J.A.; Taylor, N.F.; Brunt, R.V.; Brownsey, R.W.; Chem. Commun. 1972, 691-692.

27. Robyt, J.F. In Encyclopedia of Polymer Science and Engineering; Mark, H.F., Bikales, N.M. and Overberger, C.G., Eds.; Wiley, New York, 1986, 2nd Edition; Vol. 4, pp. 752-767.

28. Barnett, J.E.G. Biochem. J. 1971, 123, 607-611.

29. Hehre, E.J.; Brewer, C.F.; Ganghof, D.S. J. Biol. Chem. 1979, 254, 5942-5950

30. Kasumi, T.; Tsumuraya, Y.; Brewer, C.F.; Kersters-Hilderson, H.; Claeyssens, M.; Hehre, E.J. Biochemistry 1987, 26, 3010- .

31. Gold, A.M.; Osber, M.P. Biochem. Biophys. Res. Commun. 1971, 42, 469-474.

32. Treder, W.; Thiem, J.; Schlingmann, M. Tetrahedron Lett. 1986, 27, 5605-5608.

33. Sadozi, K.K.; Nukada, T.; Ito, Y.; Nakahara, Y.; Ogawa, T.; Kobata, A. Carbohydr. Res. 1986, 157, 101-123

34. Butchard, C.G.; Dwek, R.A.; Kent, P.W.; Williams, R.J.P.; Xavier, A.V. Eur. J. Biochem. 1972, 27, 548-553.

35. Hoffman, R.A.; Forsen, S.W. Progress in NMR Spectroscopy; Emsley, J.W.; Feeny, J. and Sutcliffe, Eds. Pergamon Press, Oxford, 1963, 1, 15-204.

36. Street, I.P.; Armstrong, C.R.; Withers, S.G. Biochemistry 1986, 25, 6021-6027.
37. Withers, S.G.; MacLennan, D.J.; Street, I.P. Carbohydr. Res. 1986, 154, 127-144.
38. Taylor, N.F.; Hill, L.; Eisenthal, R. Can. J. Biochem. 1975, 53, 57-64.
39. Drueckhammer, D.G.; Wong, C-H. J. Org. Chem. 1985, 50, 5912-5913.
40. Squire, S.T.; Taylor, N.F. Proc. Can. Fed. Biol. Soc. Abstr. 1985, 28, 226.
41. Brunt, R.V.; Taylor, N.F. Biochem. J. 1967, 105, 41c.
42. Brunt, R.V.; Taylor, N.F. Biochem. J. 1969, 114, 445-447.
43. Woodward, B.; Taylor, N.F.; Brunt, R.V. Biochem. Pharmacol. 1971, 20, 1071-1077.
44. Heredia, C.F.; Dela Fuente, G.; Sols, A. Biochem. Biophys. Acta 1964, 86, 216-228.
45. Miles, R.J.; Pirt, S.J.; J. Gen. Microbiol. 1973, 76, 305-318.
46. Taylor, N.F.; Louie, L.; Can. J. Biochem. 1977, 55, 911-915.
47. Peterkofsky, A.; Trends Biochem. Sci. 1977 2, 12-14.
48. White, F.H.; Taylor, N.F. FEBS Lett. 1970, 11, 268-272.
49. Midgley, M.; Dawes, E.A.; Biochem. J. 1973 132, 141-154.
50. Roberts, B.K.; Midgley, M.; Dawes, E.A. J. Gen. Microbiol. 1973, 78, 319-329.
51. Taylor, N.F.; Hill, L.; Eisenthal, R. Can. J. Biochem. 1975, 53, 57-64.
52. Entner, N.; Doudoroff, M. J. Biol. Chem. 1952, 196, 853-862.
53. D'Amore, T.; Taylor, N.F. FEBS Lett. 1982, 143, 247-251.
54. Romaschin, A.; Taylor, N.F.; Smith, D.A.; Lopes, D. Can. J. Biochem. 1977, 55, 369-375.
55. Romaschin, A.; Taylor, N.F.; Can. J. Biochem. 1981, 59, 262-268.
56. Lai, C.Y.; Horecker, B.L. in Essays in Biochemistry; Campbell, P.M. and Dicknes, F. eds. Academic Press, London, U.K. 1972, 8, p. 149.
57. Rose, J.A.; Adv. Enzymol. Relat. Areas Mol. Biol. 1975, 43, 491.
58. Agbanyo, M.; Taylor, N.F. Bioscience. Rep. 1986, 6, 309-316.
59. Defay, J.; Driguez, H.; Henrissat, B. Carbohydr. Res. 1975, 63, 41-49.
60. Wang, T.; Himoe, A. J. Biol. Chem. 1974, 249, 3895-3902.
61. Grier, T.J.; Rasmussen, J.R. Biochem. J. 1983 209, 677-685.

62. Schwarz, R.T.; Schmidt, M.F.G.; Datema, R. Biochem.
     Soc. Trans. 1979, 7, 322-326.
63. Schwarz, R.T.; Datema, R. Trends. Biochem. Sci.
     1980, 5, 65-67.
64. Hubbard, S.C.; Robbins, P.W. J. Biol. Chem. 1979,
     254, 4568-4576.
65. Datema, R.; Schwarz, R.T. Biochem. J. 1979, 184,
     113-123.
66. Datema, R.; Schwarz, R.T.; Jankowski, A.W. Eur. J.
     Biochem. 1980, 109, 331-341.
67. Datema, R.; Schwarz, R.T.; Winkler, J. Eur. J.
     Biochem. 1980, 110, 355-361.
68. McDowell, W.; Datema, R.; Romero, P.A.; Schwarz,
     R.T. Biochemistry, 1985, 24, 8145-8152.
69. Kornfeld, R.; Kornfeld, S. Ann. Rev. Biochem. 1985,
     54, 631-664.
70. Grier, T.J.; Rasmusssen, J.R. Anal. Biochem. 1982
     127, 100-104.
71. Grier, T.J.; Rasmussen, J.R. J. Biol. Chem. 1984
     259, 1027-1030.
72. Rottenberg, D.A.; Cooper, A.J.L. Trends Biochem.
     Sci. 1981, 6, 120-122.
73. Ter-Pogossian, M.M., Raichle, M.E.; Sobel, B.E. Sci.
     Amer. 1980 243, 171-181.
74. Greenberg, G.H.; Reivich, M.; Alavi, A.; Hand, P.;
     Rosequist, A.; Rintelmann, W.; Stein, A.; Tusa, R.;
     Dann, R.; Christman, D.; Fowler, J.; MacGregor, B.;
     Wolf, A. Science 1981, 212, 678-680.
75. Gallagher, B.M.; Fowler, J.S.; Gutterson, N.I.;
     MacGregory, R.R.; Wan, C.N.; Wolf, A.P. J. Nucl.
     Med. 1978, 19, 1154-1161.
76. Mizuno, T.; Kageyama, J. Biochem. 1978, 84 179-191.
77. Samuel, J.; Taylor, N.F. Carbohydr. Res. 1984, 133,
     168-172.
78. Clark, M.G. Int. J. Biochem. 1978, 9, 17-18.
79. Floridi, A. J. Chromatog. 1971, 59, 61-70.
80. Dangyan, M.T.; Arakelyan, S.V. Nauch. Trudy Esevan.
     Gosudarst. Univ. Ser. Khim., 1954, 44, 35-39; Chem.
     Abstr. 1959, 53, 21648i.
81. Janssen, F.W.; Ruelius, H.W. Biochim. Biophys. Acta
     1968, 167, 501-510.
82. Ruelius, H.W.; Kerrwin, R.M.; Janssen, F.W. Biochim.
     Biophys. Acta 1968, 167, 493-500.
83. Janssen, F.W.; Ruelius, H.W. In Methods in
     Enzymology; Wood, W.A. Ed.; Academic: New York,
     1975, 41, 170-173.'
84. Geigert, J.; Neidelman, S.L.; Hirano, D.S.
     Carbohydr. Res. 1983, 113, 159-162.
85. Geigert, J.; Neidelman, S.L.; Hirano, D.S.; Wolf,
     B.; Pauschar, B.M. Carbohydr. Res. 1983, 113, 163-
     165.
86. Yozo, M.; Toru, N. Agric. Biol. Chem. 1984, 48,
     2463-2470.

87. Lineweaver, H.; Burk, D. J. Amer. Chem. Soc. 1934, 56 568-666.
88. Eisenthal, R.; Cornish-Bowden, A. Biochem. J. 1974 139, 715-720.
89. Hanes, C.S. Biochem. J. 1932, 26, 1406-1421.
90. Hofstee, B.H.J. J. Biol. Chem. 1952, 199, 357-364.
91. Krupka, R.M. Biochem. 1966, 5 1988-1998.
92. Volo, J.; Sedmera, P.; Musilek, V. Folia Microbiol. 1978, 23, 292-298.
93. Barnett, J.E.G.; Atkins, G.R.S. Carbohydr. Res. 1972, 25, 511-515.
94. Pacak, J.; Halaskova, J.; Stepan, V.; Cerny, M. Collect. Czech. Chem. Comm. 1972, 37, 3646-3651.
95. Tipson, R.; Brady, R.F.; West, B.F. Carbohydr. Res. 1971, 16, 383-393.
96. Rao, G.V.; Que, L.; Hall, L.D.; Foudy, R.P. Carbohydr. Res. 1975, 40, 311-321.
97. Lui, F-N.E.; Wolf, B.; Geigert, J.; Neideleman, S.L.; Chin, J.D.; Hirano, D.S. Carbohydr. Res. 1983, 113, 151-157.
98. Chizov, O.S.; Kadentsev, V.I.; Zolotarev, B.M.; Foster, A.B.; Jarman, M.; Westwood, J.H. Org. Mass Spectrum 1971, 5 437-445.
99. Sharpe, A.G. in Ciba Fdn. Symp. Carbon Fluorine Compounds; Elsevier Associated Scientific Publishers, Amsterdam, 1972; 33-54.
100. Campbell-Burk, S.L.; Shulman, R.G. Ann. Rev. Microbiol. 1987, 47, 595-616.

RECEIVED January 15, 1988

Chapter 8

Sucrose Transport in Plants Using Monofluorinated Sucroses and Glucosides

William D. Hitz

Central Research and Development Department, E. I. du Pont de Nemours and Company, Experimental Station, Wilmington, DE 19898

The sucrose carrier in the outer membrane of cells of developing soybean cotyledons recognizes and transports sucrose derivitives which are singly fluorinated at C-1', C-4', and C-6'. Some $\underline{a}$-glucosides are also recognized and transported and may be used as sucrose analogs in studying carrier-substrate interaction. Phenyl $\underline{a}$-**D**-thioglucopyranosides fluorinated singly at positions C-3, C-4, and C-6 along with the deoxy-glucosides at these positions indicate that recognition by the plant carrier requires interaction at these three hydroxyls along with hydrophobic interaction with the $\underline{\beta}$-face of the glucose moiety and the $\underline{a}$-face of the fructose moiety in sucrose. 1'-Deoxy-1'-fluorosucrose is also recognized and transported by the carrier proteins in the vascular tissues of leaves and is thus moved in long distance transport in a manner identical to sucrose. At limiting substrate concentrations, 1'-deoxy-1'-fluorosucrose is metabolized by sucrose synthase at a rate 3.6 times slower than sucrose. Hydrolysis by invertase however occurs at a rate 4200 times slower than sucrose. *In vivo* rates of metabolism for the 1'-fluoro derivitive and for sucrose showed that sucrose is metabolized by both enzymes acting in parallel, and that the relative contribution of the individual enzymes varies with tissue development.

In many plant species, including virtually all major field crops and many vegetable crops, sucrose is the carbohydrate utilized

0097–6156/88/0374–0138$06.00/0

for long distance transport and for soluble, short term storage. The carbon which makes up the bulk of the dry weight harvested for economic yield is processed through the enzymes and other proteins in the physical and metabolic pathways of sucrose metabolism. Since much of the increased yield potential achieved in breeding improved varieties of crop plants has come from a more efficient transfer of carbon fixed in photosynthesis to harvestable portions of the plant (1), there is continuing interest in detailing the early steps of sucrose metabolism in order to test direct methods of improving yields through genetic or chemical modification of controlling steps in metabolism.

Two plant enzymes are capable of catalyzing the breakage of the glucose to fructose bond in sucrose. Invertase catalyzes hydrolysis either in the intra-cellular compartment or in the extra-cellular space, and sucrose synthase catalyzes the transfer of the glucose residue to Uridine diphosphate (2). Since extra-cellular invertase is present in some tissues, the membrane transport of sucrose has two possibilities also. Uptake of the intact molecule occurs as does hydrolysis followed by uptake of the hexoses produced. We have used fluorinated carbohydrates as alternate substrates for these enzymes and transport proteins in order to determine both how substrate interaction occurs and to determine which of the alternative pathways is functioning *in vivo* . The important elements of substrate interaction with carrier proteins determined from the interaction of fluorinated sucroses and sucrose analogs was used to guide the synthesis of affinity probes for protein identification and the fluorinated sucroses themselves have been used to determine the relative flux of sucrose through paralell enzymic pathways *in vivo.*

Substrate Recognition by Sucrose Transporters

Transmembrane movement of sucrose is accomplished by transport proteins in several, but not all tissue types. The most obvious example of a specific tissue type is the phloem. The sucrose concentration in this tissue can approach 0.8 M in contrast to mM concentration in the surrounding tissues and probably sub mM concentration in the extra cellular spaces surrounding the phloem (3). Transport into the cells of the phloem is difficult to study as they are an integral part of the leaf or stem structure, and may comprise only 5 to 10% of the total leaf mass. Another example of sucrose transport is the accumulation of sucrose and other nutrients by cells of developing embryos or embryo storage tissue. Large accumulations are not obvious in these tissues, but the physiological evidence suggests that sucrose uptake occurs, and that in the case of the developing soybean cotyledon, it has many of the same characteristics as phloem uptake (4.5).

Since the soybean cotyledon is quite homogeneous as to tissue type (6) and can be readily manipulated to remove cell walls in tissue slices to yield protoplasts (7), we have used these protoplasts as a model system to study membrane transport of sucrose in general. The concentration kinetics of sucrose influx suggest that at least two processes are operating in parallel. One of these is saturable with respect to sucrose concentration, of comparatively low capacity and inhibited by any of several metabolic poisons (7). The substrate specificity of this system can be studied by using alternate substrates as apparent inhibitors of the influx of radiolabled sucrose present at a concentration well below the concentration required for half-maximal uptake (K_m). Studies in which monosaccharides and natural disaccharides other than sucrose were tested as substrates show the carrier to be quite specific for sucrose (8). Accordingly, we chose to make a series of singly substituted sucroses, using fluorine as a substitute for the hydroxyl, to systematically probe the substrate binding site in the sucrose carrier protein in these cells.

Fructosyl-Substituted Sucroses.   The deoxy-fluoro-derivatives of sucrose at C-1', C-4' and C-6', along with deoxy and deoxy-azido-derivatives at   C-6' and C-1' respectively were prepared by the sucrose synthase catalyzed coupling of UDP-glucose and the substituted fructose (9.10). Those structures and their binding constants relative to sucrose (estimated from their respective K_i's) are given in Figure 1a. Substitutions at C-1' and C-6' which were more hydrophobic than the hydroxyl they replaced, bound about two fold more tightly than sucrose. The amino substitution at C-1' (formed by catalytic reduction of the 1'-azido) bound about one-half as well as the native structure. We reason that this binding pattern could occur if the three dimensional structure of sucrose associates with the binding site of the protein such that the relatively hydrophobic surface of sucrose formed by the portions of the two monosaccharide rings which are shaded in Figure 2a interact with a similarly shaped, hydrophobic site on the protein. The hydrophobic substitutions at C-1' and C-6' act to increase the size of this

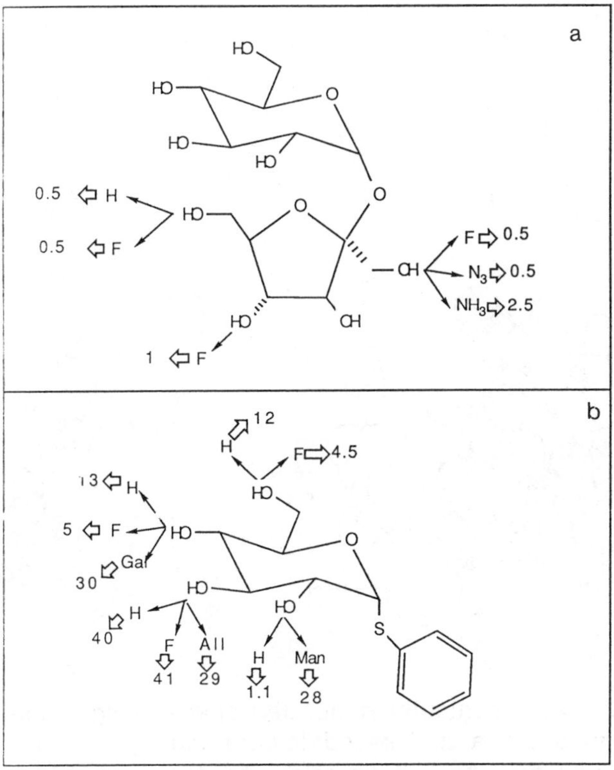

Figure 1a and 1b. The relative binding constants for 6 substituted sucroses (1a) and 10 phenyl _a_-**D**-thioglycopyranosides (1b) for the sucrose carrier protein in protoplasts derived from developing soybean cotyledons. The substrates were used as alternate substrate inhibitors of the influx of 0.2 mM ^{14}C-sucrose in an assay system described in ref. 11 . The absolute binding constant for sucrose was 2.5 mM and for phenyl _a_-**D**-thioglucopyranoside 0.35 mM. Small arrows point to the substitution and large arrows to the relative binding constant observed for that derivative. Phenyl glycosides with different sterochemistry than glucose are denoted by the three letter prefix.

A
B

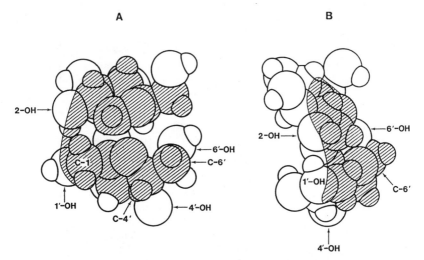

Figure 2. A, a computer generated space filling model of crystalline sucrose as viewed toward the _β_-face of the glucose ring and the _a_-face of the fructose ring. The shaded area indicates the relatively hydrophobic region, which may allow binding to a reciprocal surface on the carrier protein. B, the view of the space filling model toward the C-2 and C-1' regions showing the wedge shape of the overall structure. (Reproduced with permission from ref. 11. Copyright 1986 by the American Society of Biological Chemists, Inc.)

surface and allow greater contact with the matching protein surface. Conversely the polar, amino substitution interferes with binding and the 4'-fluoro derivative is not changed within the binding region and is thus neutral with respect to binding.

Since in this series of 5 substitutions, all but the 3'-OH of the fructose moiety of sucrose have been sequentially replaced without loss of binding, it seemed likely that the entire fructose portion of the structure might be replaced with a suitable, hydrophobic structure. In fact, phenyl *a*-D-thioglucopyranoside was shown to act as a competitive alternate substrate for sucrose influx, and the influx of phenyl [U-^{14}C]-*a*-D-thioglucopyranoside was inhibited by sucrose (11). This observation allows the use of glycosyl-substituted phenyl-thioglycopyranosides as probes for the structural requirements of the glucose portion of sucrose in binding to the carrier.

Glycosyl Substituted Thiophenyl Glycopyranosides. Alternate substrate, competition experiments were carried out using 0.2 mM ^{14}C-sucrose and concentrations of phenyl thioglucopyranoside ranging from 0.05 to 10 mM. The results are summarized in Figure 1b. Removal of the 2-OH did not reduce binding as might be expected since the 2-OH of sucrose is most likely intra-molecularly hydrogen bonded (12) and is therefore not available in ligand interactions. All modifications at C-3 resulted in essentially complete loss of binding. Assuming that fluorine is capable of hydrogen bonding as an acceptor at least to some degree, we interpret these substitutions to mean that the 3-OH donates in an essential hydrogen bonding. Inversion of the stereoconfiguration at either C-2 or C-4 resulted in complete loss of binding also; consistent with the proposed hydrophobic interaction along that surface of sucrose (Figure 2b).

Interpretation of the deoxy and deoxyfluoro substitutions at C-4 and C-6 is more difficult inasmuch as none of the four substrates either retained or lost full binding efficacy. The simplest interpretation is that hydrogen bonding does occur at both positions but that it is not an absolute requirement for recognition as it is at C-3. That the fluoro substitution at C-4 led to significantly tighter binding than the deoxy derivative may indicate that the 4-OH accepts a hydrogen bond and that fluorine is only partially effective in bonding. The results at C-4 and C-6 are also somewhat consistent with intra-molecular hydrogen bonding and recognition of the resulting surface.

There is no evidence for bonding between the 6-OH and 4-OH in sucrose however(12), and also, one of the two fluoro substitutions should have restored binding if fluorine is an effective hydrogen bond acceptor.

Substrate binding by this carrier requires the correct stereochemical placement of three closely spaced hydroxyls for recognition and the existence of a relatively hydrophobic surface of suitable shape and size. The general pattern is very similar to that described by the laboratory of Lemiex (13) for binding of carbohydrate antigens.

As a practical consequence of this work, knowledge of substrate recognition requirements has allowed the rational design of a photolyzable derivative of sucrose. Since the fructose moiety apparently resides in a hydrophobic region of the protein when sucrose is in the binding site, and since the 6'-hydroxyl is not essential for binding, that position is a good candidate for the introduction of modifications to the sucrose structure. 6'-Deoxy-6'-(4-azido-2-hydroxy)-benzamidosucrose was synthesized for utilization as a photolabile derivative of sucrose.

6'-Deoxy-6'-(4-azido-2-hydroxy)-benzamidosucrose

The modified sucrose has been shown to be a competitive inhibitor of sucrose influx into soybean cotyledon protoplasts and the phenyl ring is readily iodinated under mild conditions or by enzymic catalysis so the the photoprobe can be radiolabeled with ^{125}I. Photolysis of the labeled probe with total membrane preparations from developing soybean cotyledons produces very prominent labeling in a protein of about 62 kiloDalton (kD) molecular weight by sodium dodecyl-sulfate, polyacrylamide gel electrophoresis. The labeling is partially prevented by the inclusion of saturating concentrations of sucrose in the photolysis mixture. Cotyledons at very early stages of development do not exhibit active accumulation of sucrose and membranes prepared from tissue early in development do not contain a prominent protein of 62 kD molecular weight, and do not label at that position in photolysis experiments using the photolyzable sucrose analog.

The 62 kD integral membrane protein has been purified by differential extraction of membrane preparations with detergents, followed by ion exchange chromatography of the solubilized proteins and finally by preparative polyacrylamide gel electophoresis to obtain antigen for antibody production in rabbits. The polyclonal antibody preparations obtained are specific for the 62 kD protein using Western analysis of total protein extracts from cotyledons. Immunohistochemical analysis of cotyledon tissue at the transmission electron microscope level shows that antigen recognized by the antibody preparation is located exclusively in the outer membrane surrounding the cells. In the cotyledon, the 62 kD protein is both spatially and temporally located correctly to be a sucrose transporting protein.

Immunohistochemistry also shows that a protein which cross reacts with antibody raised against the cotyledon 62 kD protein exists in leaves. The cross reacting protein is localized primarily in three cell types of the phloem of mature leaves. Studies at the electron microscope level further show that the intra-cellular localization is again exclusively in the outer membrane of the cells. While these unpublished results do not prove that the 62 kD cotyledon protein is a sucrose carrier, they are very encouraging and may prove very useful in studying the developmental regulation of this transport process as well as providing the further tools needed to definitively identify the carrier protein.

Determination of *in vivo* Enzyme Activity

Since sucrose synthase was used to synthesize 1'-deoxy-1'-fluorosucrose (1'-FS), it must also catalyze the breakdown of 1'-FS. The work of Guthrie et. al (14) utilizing modified methyl fructofuranosides as invertase substrates, showed that hydrogen bonding (OH donating) by the 1-OH is a requirement for substrate recognition. Sucrose and 1'-FS should therefore be differentially metabolized by the two enzymes. If the appropriate kinetic parameters are known to sufficient accuracy, the relative metabolic rates for the two substrates should allow determination of the flux through both enzymes if the substrates are supplied to the enzymes functioning *in vivo*.

In vitro Kinetic Parameters.   Concentration kinetics for sucrose and 1'-FS hydrolysis by plant invertase are shown in Figure 3. The K_m for sucrose hydrolysis was about 2 mM. Hydrolysis of 1'-FS was very slow at the concentrations tested, and the data are not sufficient to determine whether both K_m and V_{max} were changed by the substitution or if only a K_m change has occurred. The data are consistent with a very high K_m for 1'-FS as would be expected if the 1'-OH were required for substrate recognition by invertase.

In contrast, sucrose synthase from wheat germ catalyzes the transfer of glucose to UDP at reasonable rates with both substrates (Figure 4).   The kinetic parameters taken from the data of Figure 4 give K_m's of 75.6 mM and 54 mM for sucrose and 1'-FS respectively.   The slower reaction rate with 1'-FS is due to a decreased maximum reaction rate (V_{max} = 52 and 15.6 nmole min^{-1}mg protein^{-1} for sucrose and 1'-FS respectively).

When substrates are used at low, radiotracer concentrations, the Michaelis-Menten equation defining reaction rate in terms of substrate concentration and enzyme kinetic parameters reduces to:

$$v = [S](V_{max}/K_m) \qquad (1)$$

where v is the reaction rate and [S] is the substrate concentration.   The relation also allows a more precise method of calculating the ratio of the kinetic constant (V_{max}/K_m) for the two substrates.   Since:

$$\frac{v_s}{v_{fs}} = \frac{[S](V_{max}/K_m}{[1'\text{-}FS](V_{max}/K_m)_{fs}} \qquad (2)$$

the ratio of products formed from a single reaction mixture containing both substrates at low concentration is equal to the ratio of substrates in the reaction times the ratio of their kinetic constants.   In practice the ratio can be determined by supplying ^{3}H-sucrose and [14]C-1'-FS in varying ratios, stopping the reaction after conversion of a very small amount of substrate and determining the ^{3}H to ^{14}C ratio in the common product, UDP-glucose.   The results of such an experiment are

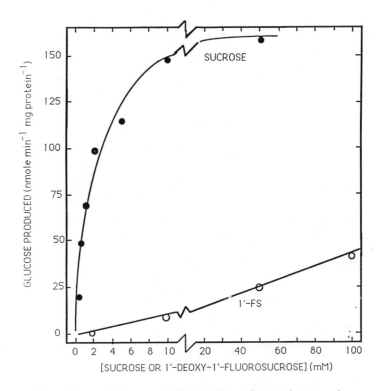

Figure 3. The substrate concentration dependence of sucrose or 1'-deoxy-1'-fluorosucrose hydrolysis by invertase from developing leaves of sugarbeet. Invertase activity was assayed at pH 5 by measuring glucose production as described in ref. 16.

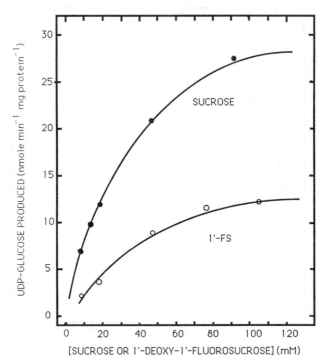

Figure 4. The substrate concentration dependence of the rate of UDP-glucose production from either sucrose or 1'-deoxy-1'-fluorosucrose and UDP by sucrose synthase. Sucrose synthase was partially purified from wheat germ and UDP-glucose production was assayed as described in ref. 16.

shown in Figure 5 and give a ratio of kinetic constants of 3.6; very similar to that obtained from the ratio of the four components determined individually.

Similar experiments done with invertase hydrolysis of the two substrates at ratios appropriate to allow analysis of the product, in spite of the large difference in reaction rates gives a ratio of about 4200 for the same kinetic parameters.

Relative Activities of Invertase and Sucrose Synthase *in vivo*. Developing plant leaves are supplied with sucrose by older leaves until they become photosynthetically competent.   Such developing leaves have extractable activity in both sucrose cleaving enzymes (15).   To determine the relative flux through the two enzymes in developing soybean leaves, tracer quantities of [U-^{14}C]-a -**D**-glucopyranosyl β -**D**-fructofuranoside (glucosyl-^{14}C-sucrose) and [U-^{14}C]-a -**D**-glucopyranosyl β-**D**-1-deoxy-1-fluoro-fructofuranoside (glucosyl-^{14}C-1'FS) were supplied to a mature leaf by perfusing an abrasion on the leaf surface with a buffered solution containing one of the sugars. Arrival of label in the developing leaflets was monitored with a Geiger-Mueller tube (16).   The rate of arrival of label from both sugars was identical Figure 6), indicating very similar rates of transport for both tracers.

Since the first step in sucrose metabolism must be one of the two   (enzymes, the rate of ^{14}C arrival in any product of glucose metabolism is a measure of the combined flux through the two sucrose metabolism paths.   For simplicity of analysis therefore, developing leaf tissue samples were taken, label soluble in 80% ethanol was extracted to remove unreacted sucrose or 1'-FS, and the label incorporated into insoluble products of glucose metabolism was determined.   Figure 7 shows time courses for conversion of imported label to insoluble products from the two sugars in carbon importing leaves at various stages of development.

Rates of metabolism can be determined for each sugar from the experimental time period in which incorporation into insolubles is   linear. Rates of metabolism determined in this way change with leaf development.   The metabolism rate for both sugars increases during early development and then declines, however the rate of sucrose metabolism increases more than the rate of 1'-FS metabolism over the same developmental period.   This indicates a changing relative contribution by the two sucrose metabolizing enzymes.

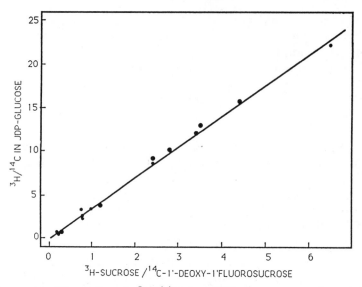

Figure 5. The ratio of $^3H/^{14}C$ in UDP-glucose produced from incubation of varying ratios of ^3H-sucrose to ^{14}C-1'-deoxy-1'-fluorosucrose with UDP and sucrose synthase purified from developing soybean leaves as described in ref. 16.

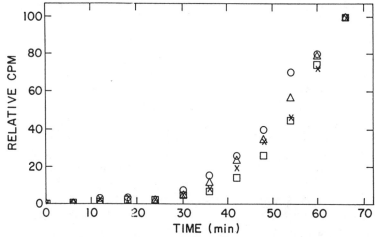

Figure 6.   Translocation of ^{14}C-sucrose (x,□) and ^{14}C-1'-deoxy-1'-fluorosucrose (Δ, O) into young soybean leaves. Counts per minute (CPM), measured by Geiger-Mueller counting, were corrected for background and expressed as per cent of CPM at 66 min. ^{14}C-sugars were supplied to an exporting leaf at time zero by application of a buffered solution containing the sugar to an abraded surface. (Reproduced with permission from ref. 16. Copyright 1987 The American Society of Plant Physiologists.)

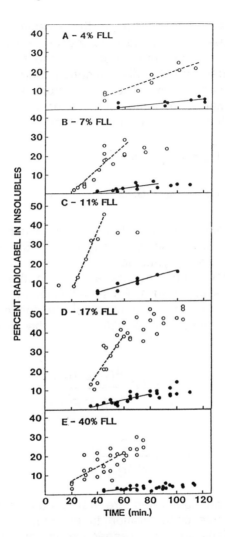

Figure 7.   The time course of percent incorporation into ethanol insolubles of phloem translocated sucrose (o) and 1'-deoxy-1'-fluorosucrose (•) in soybean first trifoliolate leaves of various ages (%FLL is the percent of final leaf length of a comparable leaf at maturity).   Radiolabled sucrose and/or 1'-deoxy-1'-fluorosucrose were supplied as described in Figure 3 and importing leaves were either removed from sampling at time points or parts of the leaf were removed at time points and extracted as described in the text.   (Reproduced with permission from ref. 16.   Copyright 1987 The American Society of Plant Physiologists.)

Quantitative determination of the relative contributions of sucrose synthase and invertase to the breakdown of phloem-supplied sucrose can be determined from the total metabolism rate for each sugar and the discrimination factor for the two sugars as substrates for invertase and sucrose synthase. The total rate of breakdown of either sucrose or 1'-FS is the sum of the fluxes through the two enzymes so that:

$$R_S = I_S + SS_S \qquad (3)$$

$$\text{and} \quad R_{fs} = I_{fs} + SS_{fs} \qquad (4)$$

where R is the total rate of metabolism for either sugar, I is the contribution of invertase to that rate, and SS is the contribution of sucrose synthase.

At the tracer concentrations arriving in the importing leaf, the ratio of sucrose to 1'-FS metabolism by sucrose synthase is 3.6 times the ratio of substrate concentration, and the same ratio for invertase is 4200 times the ratio of substrate concentration. Thus:

$$SS_S = 3.6\ SS_{fs} \frac{[^{14}C\text{-sucrose}]}{[^{14}C\text{-}1'\text{-FS}]} \qquad (5)$$

$$\text{and} \quad I_S = 4200\ I_{fs} \frac{[^{14}C\text{-sucrose}]}{[^{14}C\text{-}1'\text{-FS}]} \qquad (6)$$

Since the two substrates are transported identically, and supplied at the same concentration to the mature leaves, their initial concentrations in their respective importing leaves will be very similar and the substrate ratios in equations 5 and 6 will be essentially one. Since sucrose is always metabolized faster than 1'-FS, the ratio will become less than one with time and the apparent relative metabolism rates for the two sugars will change as can be seen in figure 7. During the initial, linear period of label incorporation into insolubles however the ratio can be assumed to be one. Assuming this simplification, dividing equation 3 by equation 4 and substituting for SS_{fs} and I_{fs} from equations 5 and 6 respectively, then solving for I_S/SS_S, gives

$$I_S/SS_S = \frac{1-(Rs/Rfs)/3.6}{(Rs/Rfs)4200-1}$$

The ratios R_S/R_{fS} from the data of figure 7 and the corresponding contributions of invertase and sucrose synthase calculated from those ratios are given in Table I for leaves of different developmental ages.

Table I. The relative contribution of invertase and sucrose synthase to sucrose metabolism in developing soybean leaves

Leaf Age	Rate of Sugar Metabolism [b]				% of Total Metabolism	
(% FLL)[a]	_Rs_	_Rfs_	_Rs/Rfs_	_Is/SSs_[c]	_Is_	_SSs_
4.0	0.25	0.074	3.4	0	0	100
7.6	0.64	0.095	6.7	0.86	46	54
11.0	1.5	0.19	7.9	1.20	54	46
17.0	1.0	0.16	6.2	0.72	42	58
40.0	0.37	0.059	6.5	0.75	43	57

[a]Leaf age as determined by the % of length attained by a comparable leaf   at full development.
[b]Rate of sucrose or 1'-FS metabolism in % of total radiolabel in the leaf converted to insolubles per minute.
[c]Calculated using equation 7.

The rate of carbon import and sucrose metabolism increased very rapidly during early development. Most of the increased rate of sucrose metabolism could be accounted for by a sharp rise in the flux through invertase. As the leaf became photosynthetically competent, the rate of utilization of carbon imported from mature leaves declined, however about one-half of sucrose metabolism remained through invertase.

In leaves at early stages of development, extractable invertase activity (measured at its pH optima) can exceed extractable sucrose synthase activity by 10 to 20 fold (15), yet compartmentalization of enzyme and substrate may make the relative flux through these parallel paths quite different from the proportionate activities.   The method described above is one of the few that can discern *in vivo* flux in this way.   As a general method it could be applied to any system for which differentially metabolizable substrates can be produced.   In the case of 1'-FS used in this way, a problem arises due to the extreme discrimination against 1'-FS by invertase.   A very small change in the ratio R_S/R_{fs} corresponds to a large change in the flux through invertase, making the calculation very sensitive to errors in the ratio.

Conclusions and Future Studies

The tenative identification of a sucrose carrier protein opens many avenues of research including the identification of sucrose binding proteins in other tissues using the sucrose photoprobe and utilizing antibody cross reactivity.   Ultimately the function of the 62 kD membrane protein from cotyledons needs to be proven either by the biochemical methods of reconstitution into artificial membrane vesicles, by comparison of the implied protein structure (obtained from the structural gene sequence) with other, known transporters, or by genetically manipulating transport.

The use of fluorinated sucroses as tracers of sucrose metabolism in order to differentiate between glycolysis started by invertase and glycolysis started by sucrose synthase should be quite useful in determining the *in vivo* flux of these paths and the large differences in phosphate metabolism which accompany the two routes of carbon metabolism.

Acknowledgments

The active collaborations of Dr. Peter Card in the synthesis of fluorinated carbohydrates, Mr. Kevin Ripp in protein purification and preparation of antibodies, Dr. Vincent Francheschi in immunohistochemistry and Dr. Judy Schmalstig in the metabolism of 1'-deoxy-1'-flurosucrose are greatfully acknowledged.

Literature Cited

1.   Gifford, R. M.; Thorne, J.; Hitz, W.; Giaquinta, R. Science 1984, 225, 801-8.

2. Avigad, G. In Plant Carbohydrates I. Encyclopedia of Plant Physiology. New Series; Springer-Verlag: Berlin, 1982; vol. 13A; pp. 217-347.
3. Giaquinta, R. T. In The Biochemistry of Plants; Academic: New York, 1980; vol. 3; pp. 271-320.
4. Lichtner, F. T.; Spanswick, R. Plant Physiol. 1981, 68, 693-8.
5. Thorne, J. H. Plant Physiol. 1982, 70,953-8.
6. Thorne, J. H. Plant Physiol. 1981, 67, 1016-25.
7. Lin, W.; Schmitt, M.; Hitz, W.; Giaquinta, R. Plant Physiol. 1984, 75, 936-40.
8. Schmitt, M. R.; Hitz, W.; Lin, W.; Giaquinta, R. Plant Physiol. 1984, 75, 941-6
9. Card, P. J.; Hitz, W. J. Am. Chem. Soc. 1984, 106, 5348-50.
10. Card, P. J.; Hitz, W. J. Am. Chem. Soc. 1986, 108, 158-61.
11. Hitz, W. D.; Card, P.; Ripp, K. J. Biol. Chem. 1986, 261, 11986-91.
12. Mathlouthi, M.; Cholli, A.; Koenig, J. Carbo. Res. 1986, 147, 1-9.
13. Hindsgual, O.; Norberg, T.; Lependu, J.; Lemeiux, R. Carbo. Res. 1982, 109.109-142.
14. Guthrie, R. D.; Jenkins, I.; Yamasaki, R. Aust. J. Chem. 1982, 35, 1003-8.
15. Giaquinta, R. T. Plant Physiol. 1978, 61, 380-5.
16. Schmalstig, J. G.; Hitz, W. Plant Physiol. 1987, 85, 407-12.

RECEIVED January 15, 1988

Chapter 9

Preparation of Fluorine-18 Deoxyfluorohexoses for Metabolism and Transport Studies

S. John Gatley[1], James E. Holden[2], Timothy R. DeGrado[2], Chin K. Ng[2], James R. Halama[2], and Robert A. Koeppe[2]

[1]The University of Chicago, Franklin McLean Institute, Box 433, 5841 South Maryland Avenue, Chicago, IL 60637
[2]Medical Physics Department, University of Wisconsin, 1300 University Avenue, Madison, WI 53706

The preparation of deoxyfluorohexoses labeled with the positron emitter Fluorine-18, and their use in studies of hexose transport and phosphorylation with isolated perfused working rat hearts is described. Compartmental analysis methods were applied to time courses of F-18, measured with scintillation probes, in hearts given 2-deoxy-2-fluoro-D-glucose (2FDG). Rate constants determined from model fits were used to calculate 2FDG distribution volumes and phosphorylation rates for hearts operated without insulin at two work loads and several perfusate glucose concentrations. Estimates of intracellular glucose contents were made from the F-18 data and independent measures of glucose utilization. The results confirm the saturability of glucose transport with increasing perfusate glucose and showed enhanced glucose content at higher workloads.

The growing interest in sugars labeled with Fluorine-18 over the last dozen years has been fuelled by the development of positron emission tomography (PET) as a medical imaging modality (1). The concentration of a radionuclide which decays with emission of a positron can be measured accurately within the human body, by coincidence detection of the pair of 511keV gamma rays which are created when each positron and an atomic electron are mutually annihilated. Commercial tomographs are now available with a spatial resolution of about 5mm, and with suitable radiotracers the rates of metabolic and physiological processes can be estimated in the brains and other organs of patients and experimental subjects. PET is distinguished from routine, clinical nuclear medical imaging by its superior quantitation and spatial isolation. In addition, an accident of nature has decreed that the longest lived externally detectable isotopes of the most

0097–6156/88/0374–0156$06.00/0

important biological elements, oxygen, nitrogen, and carbon, are all positron emitters. Thus, imaging based on positron annihilation radiation is most appropriate for *in vivo* studies with a majority of metabolically active compounds. There are no isotopes of hydrogen which emit gamma rays or positrons, but fluorine can often substitute for hydrogen (or hydroxyl groups) with retention of biological activity, and F-18 is a readily available nuclide with an extremely convenient half-life (110 minutes) for *in vivo* medical use. Short as this half-life may appear to workers accustomed to conventional biomedical tracers with half-lives ranging from weeks to millenia, recent developments have made it possible to prepare many F-18 compounds in high yields based on the isotope (2). The other important positron emitters, C-11, N-13, and O-15, in fact have considerably shorter half-lives of 20, 10, and 2 minutes respectively (3). F-18 has two other advantages apart from its half-life. One is that it is available, in moderate activities, from nuclear reactors, as well as from cyclotrons (or other charged-particle accelerators) (4). O-15, N-13, and C-11 are only available from cyclotrons. The second advantage is that the range of the positron in tissue (about 2mm) is shorter than for the other nuclides, so that higher resolution images are in principle available, although the state-of-the-art in tomograph design does not yet make this important.

The most important organic PET radiotracer is 2-deoxy-2-fluoro-D-glucose (5), which is abbreviated to 2FDG by workers in this field, probably because the tracer kinetic theory underlying its use is that developed by Sokoloff's group for animal autoradiographic studies with C-14 2-deoxy-D-glucose, which is commonly termed 2DG (6). Thus, the abbreviation 2FDG carries with it the implication that its distribution can be interpreted in the same way as that of 2DG. The rationale of the 2(F)DG method is the isolation of the hexokinase reaction which occurs because the resulting 2(F)DG-6-phosphate is structurally incapable of taking part in the subsequent hexose-6-phosphate isomerase reaction of the normal glycolytic pathway (7). The phosphorylated tracer is said to be metabolically trapped (8), since dephosphorylation is very slow in most tissues, such as brain (9), while direct diffusion out of the cell or metabolism to more diffusible species do not occur to significant extents. The amount of 2(F)DG-6-P accumulated can be determined from the total radioactivity in each brain region, by applying a tracer kinetic model (6,10). Local rates of glucose metabolism are then estimated from the known proportionality between glucose and 2(F)DG phosphorylation rates (11). Extensive discussion of these aspects of the 2(F)DG method can be found in the cited references.

Preparation of F-18 Fluorosugars

The preparation of reactive F-18 has recently been reviewed (4). Labeled molecular fluorine was first prepared from the ^{20}Ne(d, alpha)^{18}F reaction by bombarding Ne-20 containing a trace of F_2 with a deuteron beam in an all-nickel cyclotron target (12). Approximately one third of the radioisotope is exchanged into the desired chemical form, the rest being either bound to the nickel surface or in unreactive F-18 gases. Later technical developments allowed the use of a proton beam via the $^{18}O(p,n)^{18}F$ nuclear reaction (13). Techniques were also developed for conveniently converting F-18 F_2 into the more selective fluorinating agents, CH_3CO_2F and XeF_2 (14-16). A parallel developmental process has occurred with production of F-18 fluoride ion and with reaction conditions for displacement reactions. There are many nuclear reactions which lead to F-18, but the most convenient of these produce the nuclide as aqueous solutions of fluoride. These tended to be avoided a decade ago, in part because it was recognized that fluoride takes a long time to dry. In fact, yields obtained from nucleophilic substitution reactions of F-18 fluoride at that time tended to be low (17). However, this was probably due to the use of poorly reactive starting materials, inhibitory contaminants of F-18 solutions and sub-optimal reaction conditions, as much as to the presence of water. Conditions for successful nucleophilic displacement reactions leading to F-18 fluorosugars involve: a polar aprotic solvent, usually acetonitrile which has the useful property of forming a low boiling azeotrope with water (18); a supporting salt, which consists of a large easily dehydrated cation like tetraethylammonium and a basic anion such as hydroxide, which probably pulls water from fluoride ions (19), and a reactive leaving group such as triflate or cyclic sulfate. In practice, 5-50 micromole of supporting salt is added to the aqueous solution of F-18, which is then evaporated to dryness in vacuo or in a stream of nitrogen. Starting material is then added, in stoichiometric quantity with the supporting salt, with 1-10mL of acetonitrile. Incorporation reactions are generally complete in a few minutes at reflux temperature (20). Higher yields are often obtained with potassium plus Kryptofix 2,2,2 rather than a tetraalkylammonium cation (21). This may be because the aminopolyether can also encrypt traces of cations, derived from the cyclotron target, which bind fluoride tightly. A less basic cation than hydroxide, such as carbonate, may also increase yields when a base sensitive protective group, like acetate, is present in the starting material. The use of potassium/Kryptofix is not necessary if the F-18 is purified via fluorotrimethylsilane (22). This is easily generated by reaction of a crude F-18 fluoride solution with chlorotrimethylsilane and can be swept out of the reaction vessel in a stream of air. After scrubbing the gas can be cryotrapped for subsequent hydrolysis, or directly converted to fluoride by bubbling the gas stream through aqueous acetonitrile containing tetraethylammonium hydroxide. This procedure takes only about five minutes and is virtually quantitative. It separates the F-18 from traces of elements which otherwise tie up added fluoride with electrostatic or covalent bonds under the conditions used for the substitution reaction.

Routes to 2FDG

The preparation of 2FDG has been approached from both electrophilic and nucleophilic F-18 intermediates (23). The first reported route employed addition of F-18 labeled molecular fluorine (0.1-1% F_2 diluted with Ne) across the 1,2 double bond in 3,4,6-triacetylglucal (24). Addition occurs predominantly, but not exclusively, to give the glucose derivative; about one quarter of the F_2 adds to give the 2-deoxy-2-fluoro mannosyl fluoride. Greater stereospecificity is achieved using F-18 acetylhypofluorite with about 5% of the mannose compound being produced under optimal conditions (25,26). In contrast, direct F-18 fluorination of glucal in water gives a higher proportion of the mannose compound (27-29). Xenon difluoride labeled with F-18 has also been used to fluorinate triacetylglucal (30,31). While optimization of fluorinating agent and reaction conditions greatly improved the yield of 2FDG, these electrophilic syntheses were intrinsically less efficient than desired because the F_2 and CH_3CO_2F are themselves produced in poor yield (32-34). It was early recognized that a nucleophilic displacement reaction involving F-18 fluoride anion would offer improved stereospecificity and greater yield, but several years passed before successful starting materials and reaction conditions were developed.

Tewson's use of 1-beta-O-methyl-4,6-benzylidene-D- mannose 2,3-cyclic sulfate provided the first practicable nucleophilic synthesis of 2FDG (35,36). The corresponding 1-alpha-O-methyl compound failed to give good incorporation yields, but the 2-fluoro-beta-O-methyl product was difficult to deprotect. Boron tris(trifluoroacetate) in trifluoroacetic acid gave adequate yields of 2FDG, and HPLC (aminopropyl column with 70% acetonitrile) showed a small impurity peak which was ascribed to residual beta-methyl 2FDG. Subsequent experience demonstrated that the situation was more complicated. HPLC analyses in reaction mixtures revealed two peaks of roughly equal size and at least three small impurity peaks after deprotection and de-salting (37). Futhermore, in our hands the yield of 2FDG in the deprotection step was always close to 50%, and most of the remaining F-18 behaved like fluoride. It thus appears that only half the organic label in reaction mixtures is protected 2FDG. The other half is largely decomposed to HF by boron tris (trifluoroacetate). Whether this fraction is the product of nucleophilic attack at C-3, or of a rearrangement reaction of the protected 2FDG is not at present clear. The related beta-O-vinyl starting material (38) deprotects easily with 2N-HCl, but also gives a final product with several percent of labeled impurities.

A starting material with a triflate group on C-2 of a protected mannose (4,6-benzylidene-2-triflylsulfonyl-3-O-methyl-beta-O-methyl-D-mannose) was first reported by Elmaleh et al (39). Good incorporation was achieved, but the 3-O-methyl group proved impossible to remove efficiently under the time constraints of working with F-18. Synthesis of the analogous 3-O-benzyl compound was later reported (40). The current starting material of choice for nucleophilic 2FDG production is 1,3,4,6-tetra-acetyl-2-O-triflyl-D mannose (41). This incorporates F-18 rapidly in high yield from preparations of reactive F-18 fluoride, and the tetraacetyl 2FDG is cleanly deprotected by 1N-HCl. Net yields of around 50% are obtained in 45 minutes starting with an aqueous

solution of F-18 fluoride. F-18 2FDG has also been produced in low
yield by epoxide cleavage with labeled KHF$_2$ in 1,2-anhydro-3,4:5,
6-di-O-isopropylidene-1-C-nitro-D mannitol (42).

Other F-18 Sugars.

Since a wide range of F-18 reactive intermediates is now
available, any published synthesis of a fluorocarbohydrate can in
principle be adapted to use the radioisotope. The synthesis must
be completed within at most an hour or two, which necessitates
considerable attention to the rate of each step which occurs after
incorporation of the isotope. This incorporation step should be
as late in the synthetic scheme as possible. Christman et al. (43)
investigated the influence of several reaction parameters on the
synthesis of 6-deoxy 6-fluoro-D-galactose. They used a labeled
tetraalkylammonium fluoride solution in acetonitrile to displace
a variety of leaving groups in the 6-position of
1,2-3,4-diisopropylidenegalactose. Yields were rather low. The
similar synthesis of F-18 3-deoxy-3-fluoro-D-glucose (44-46)
(3FDG) from 1,2-5,6-diisopropylidene allose employed the more
reactive triflate group instead of the tosyl group originally used
for unlabeled 3FDG by Foster et al (47). Incorporation of
fluoride from tetraethylammonium fluoride was found to be complete
in a few minutes in refluxing acetonitrile (20), whereas 48 hours
(47) was allowed for reaction with the tosylate. Papers featuring
F-18 3FDG have appeared in the nuclear medicine (48) and
physiology (49) literature. It is a good substrate for glucose
transport, but a poor substrate for hexokinase (50) and has been
used to study local rates of glucose transport in PET experiments
(51). This is in contrast to studies with 2FDG which give local
rates of glucose phosphorylation. As mentioned above, the
electrophilic syntheses of 2FDG yield 3,4,6-triacetyl-2-deoxy-2-
fluoro-D-mannosyl fluoride or the corresponding 1-acetyl compound
as a side product. This can be separated and deprotected to give
2-deoxy-2-fluoro-D-mannose (2FDM) (52) though yields are poor and
it is difficult to avoid contamination with 2FDG. The
corresponding problem of 2FDG preparations containing variable
amounts of 2FDM has caused considerable anxiety in the PET
community. Although 2FDM, like 2FDG, is a good substrate for both
transport and phosphorylation, the relative rates of the epimers
for the two processes are almost certainly different, and
contamination with 2FDM will, therefore, cause erroneous values of
glucose metabolic rate to be calculated in 2FDG studies. The two
sugars are hard to separate chromatographically, so that the
severity of the problem in each batch of fluorosugar is not easy
to determine. Just as the nucleophilic routes to 2FDG do not
produce 2FDM as a contaminant, a nucleophilic pathway which is
reported to give pure 2FDM is now available. The starting material
is beta-O-methyl-4,6-benzylidene-3-O-benzyl-2-O- triflyl-D-
glucopyranose (53). Incorporation of F-18 proceeds readily, but
the product requires quite vigorous conditions (5N-HCl under
reflux for 30 minutes) for deprotection (54).
    Figure 1 shows the structures of several of the starting
materials used in syntheses of fluorosugars from F-18 fluoride.

Included is 2,3,6-tribenzoyl-4-triflyl alpha-methyl-D-galactoside which we are examining as a precursor of F-18 4-deoxy-4-fluoro-D-glucose: nucleophilic substitution has occurred readily to give a single product in most test reactions, but partial deprotection has been seen in some. We are presently optimizing conditions for controlled removal of the protective groups from the incorporation product.

Some tumors contain large quantities of L-fucose. This encouraged the development of 2-deoxy-2-fluoro-L-fucose as a potential imaging agent for detecting and monitoring such malignancies (55). The route involved addition of electrophilic F-18 to diacetyl fucal in glacial acetic acid or Freon 11.

Rapid Purfication and Quality Control

There are several significant practical differences between the preparation of compounds labeled with isotopes of very short half-lives, and traditional organic synthesis. These include: the need for radiation protection; the small scale; the need for great speed; that yields are based on the inorganic radionuclide rather than the organic starting material; some simple, yet powerful methods such as recrystallization and melting point determination cannot be applied. Clearly, a fresh batch of any F-18 sugar has to be prepared on at least a daily basis, and the term "quality control" reflects this.

Batches of F-18 sugars are typically prepared using a few milligrams of organic precursor, while the starting radioactivity of F-18 may be anything up to 1 Curie. Electrophilic F-18 fluorinations are generally performed with tens of micromoles of carrier fluorine. In contrast, for nucleophilic F-18 fluorinations the mass of fluorine is generally tiny, consisting of the F-18 itself (about 0.6 nanomole per Curie) plus any non-radioactive F-19 present in reagents, which is usually of the order of 1 nanomole. These are referred to as "no carrier added" conditions. The labeled product then has a very high specific radioactivity, which circumvents any possible toxic or pharmacologic effects during human use. The overall scale of both electrophilic and nucleophilic reactions is small enough to allow analytical methodologies to be used preparatively during work-up and purification. For example, acids used in deprotection can be removed by passage through small columns of ion-retardation resin. Traces of F-18 fluoride are removed with alumina columns, and unhydrolyzed initial labeled products, if neutral, are retained on octadecylsilane bonded silica gel. Objectionable color may often be removed with activated charcoal, and sterilization achieved with a 0.2 micron Millipore filter. Labeled reaction products not held up in this cascade of absorbents and filters would include alkylglycosides and neutral rearrangement products. Most of the starting materials for fluoride based synthesis of deoxyfluoro sugars yield the corresponding parent sugar, originating from nucleophilic attack of hydroxide ion or water, as the dominant unlabeled impurity. Because of the small amount of starting material, the concentration of unlabeled material is not objectionable for PET work. For example, glucose in human blood plasma is present at about 5 micromole/mL in about 5L of fluid; thus vascular injection of 5ml of 2FDG preparation containing 10-20 micromole of glucose does not perturb glucose homeostasis. For work with isolated organs (see below), however, the injectate must be free of glucose and other unlabeled impurities.

The method of choice for preparative separation of desired F-18 fluorosugar from either labeled or unlabeled impurities is high performance liquid chromatography (HPLC), and this is also the most common option for quality control. Two popular stationary phases are aminopropyl derivatized silica and certain cation exchange resins. The former is cheaper and easier to use, but the latter has superior resolution for many sugars and has the advantage for preparative use of using water as mobile phase rather than aqueous acetonitrile. Fluoride ion and some other compounds have very long retention times in both types of HPLC column, and it is easy to overestimate the radiochemical purities of fluorosugars by failure to notice very broad late running peaks. Thin layer chromatography (TLC) has inferior resolution to HPLC but the advantage that labeled spots close to the origin are as easily detected on autoradiographs as compounds with large RF values. Another analytical strategy for some F-18 fluorosugars is to compare chromatograms before and after using hexokinase plus ATP/Mg^{2+} to generate the 6-phosphates (56). Figure 2 shows a chromatogram of a preparation of 2FDG made from the beta-methyl cyclic sulfate starting material. In this case there is a small labeled impurity co-eluting with 2FDG on the amino column, which is demonstrated by the residual peak left after treatment with hexokinase. This illustrates a potential problem in relying on retention time alone, or in a single system, for quality control. The 2FDG-6-phosphate is retained on the column indefinitely under these conditions. The sugar phosphates can also be easily trapped with anion exchange resins and the phosphorylatable fraction of a preparation determined.

Application of F-18 Fluorosugars

Syntheses of several F-18 fluorosugars have now been developed to the point at which they can easily be prepared on a small scale where radiation exposure is not a serious issue (say, up to 1 mCi) in any laboratory situated within several hours of a suitable nuclear reactor (57) or accelerator. Molecular and biological scientists can, therefore, consider working with this isotope. One advantage is that F-18 is easily detected and counted quantitatively, in any kind of sample, without the tedious preparation needed for C-14 or tritium; the time saved more than compensates for the need to prepare the F-18 tracer every day. Another is the extremely high specific radioactivity obtainable, which allows a tracer state (i.e., no perturbation of the system under study) to be maintained, and which permits slow processes and binding sites present in low concentrations to be investigated.

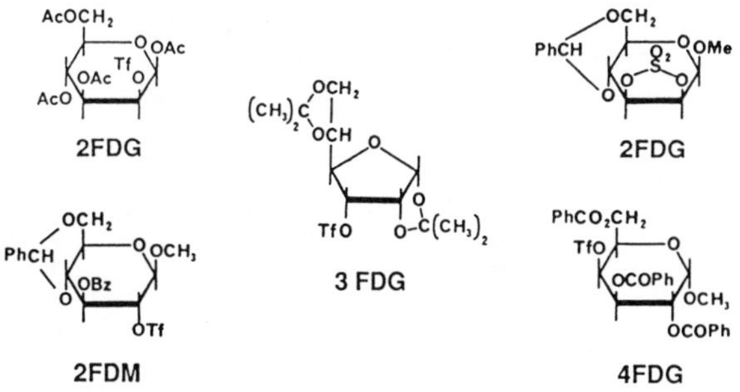

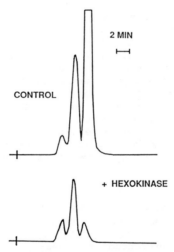

Figure 1. Structures of precursors for nucleophilic routes to deoxyfluorohexoses.

Figure 2. High performance liquid chromatogram of a preparation of 2-deoxy-2-fluoro-D-glucose. Stationary phase, aminopropyl banded silica; mobile phase, 70% aqueous acetonitrile at 1.5mL/min. The large peak in the upper panel is 2FDG.

Animal Experiments

Data from experiments (32,49) in which three F-18 sugars were injected into rats are shown in Table I.

TABLE I. Tissue-to-blood ratios of D-2FDG,
D-3FDG and L-3FDG in rats at 60 min

Organ	D-2FDG	D-3FDG	L-3FDG
Brain	6.22±1.2	0.82±0.25	0.13±0.12
Heart	12.9±5.6	1.17±0.47	0.69±0.17
Kidney	4.38±4.3	1.43±0.63	3.59±1.67
Liver	1.28±0.09	0.90±0.31	0.80±0.23
Muscle	0.71±0.17	0.53±0.29	0.47±0.23
Urine	40-60%	5-20%	50-60%

The distribution of the unnatural L-3FDG, which we expect to be neither a substrate for transport systems, nor to be metabolized, is consistent with its being largely confined to the extracellular fluid, and its rapid elimination via the kidneys. The brain, with its tight capillary structure, particularly excludes L-3FDG. A strikingly different picture is given by D-3FDG, with much less F-18 in urine and more F-18 in brain and heart. This behavior confirms that D-3FDG is specifically transported in several tissues, and the relative accumulation seen in heart hints at a specific trapping mechanism. Much greater tissue-to-blood ratios in heart and brain were seen in animals given D-2FDG, which is not only transported into these organs, but is trapped as the 6-phosphate to a greater degree than D-3FDG. However, D-2FDG is not, unlike D-3FDG, a substrate for the energy-linked carrier in the kidney tubules, and so is eliminated faster. This is an advantage in whole body imaging studies, because it causes the "background" due to F-18 in blood to decrease rapidly.

Isolated Perfused Hearts

Differences in the behavior of D-2FDG, D-3FDG and L-3FDG were seen more clearly when they were administered to isolated perfused rat hearts (49) (Figure 3). Briefly, 10 microliters of tracer in perfusion medium was presented in a nearly instantaneous (<0.25 seconds) bolus into the coronary arteries of a heart in metabolic steady state. A specially designed coincidence counting system, based on cesium fluoride crystal scintillators, and capable of measuring the radioactivity remaining in the organ over the range 100 microCuries to 1 nanoCurie, was constructed for these experiments (58). The appearance of residue curves for the three fluorosugars was very similar at times up to 1 minute after the time of maximum count rate. This is because most of the F-18 at early times is in the extracellular pools, and behaves in much the same way for each compound. After 1 minute the residue curves become easily distinguishable; each has a "tail", but about an

order of magnitude separates D-2FDG from D-3FDG and the latter
from its stereoisomer. Presumably, the tail for L-3FDG and its
slow clearance represents slow non-carrier mediated diffusion into
and out of heart cells. The behavior of the D sugars, however,
suggests formation and slow hydrolysis of their 6-phosphates. The
larger tail for 2FDG than for 3FDG, is reasonable, because the
former is a much better substrate for hexokinase (50), so that
more 2FDG-6-phosphate than 3FDG-6-phosphate can be synthesized
during the early period when the cellular concentration of
fluorosugar is high.   These early experiments with isolated
perfused hearts gave results which were interpretable mainly
qualitatively. The development of the method to the point of
giving quantitative information and thus providing a new window on
physiological processes has taken several years. In addition to
the development of the radiochemistry and the counting system, it
was necessary to learn to maintain hearts at physiological work
loads and in metabolic steady state. We adapted the perfusion
system of Taegtmeyer (59). Also, the experiments required
apparatus and techniques for gathering ancillary physiological and
biochemical information. Finally, the work necessitated
implementation of computer fitting routines for compartmental
analysis of the residue curves. The routine finds the best set of
rate-constants which describe each curve. The approach of Chu and
Berman (60) was used here, modified for use with a mini-computer
(61).

The compartmental model used for 2FDG, comprising five
compartments and rate constants describing transfer between them,
is shown in Figure 4. We have evaluated several other models, but
none gives as good fits to residue curves. For example, Figure 5
shows data for the very early portion of an experiment, together
with a fit (dashed line) to the model of Figure 4 which clearly
matches the points very well. Values of chi-squared are always
close to 1.00. The solid line in Figure 5 is the best fit obtained
using basically the same model, but treating the interstitial and
cellular free tracer as one compartment instead of two. Although
data are well fitted at later times, they are poorly fitted in the
first half minute, when rapid filling of the interstitium and
slower transfer to the cellular pool are occurring. Chi-squared
values of around 1.20 are obtained when this simplified model is
used.

Some of the rate constants, and combinations of them, have
important physiological meaning, for example: k^*_{32} describes the
carrier mediated transport of 2FDG from the interstitium into the
cells; $k^*_{32}/(k^*_{23} + k^*_{43})$ is the equilibrium ratio of the cellular
and interstitial distribution volumes of the tracer; k^*_{43} describes
the operation of hexokinase; $k^*_{32} \cdot k^*_{43}/(k^*_{23} + k^*_{43})$ is
proportional to the phosphorylation rate of 2FDG, and k^*_{34} is the
rate-constant for hydrolysis of the 6-phosphate of 2FDG.   Thus
several aspects of fluorosugar behavior can be measured with a
single injection of tracer.   It is vitally important before
drawing inferences from kinetic radioactivity data to thoroughly
understand the metabolism of the tracer. The model to which the
residue curves are fitted (Figure 4) assumes the existence of two

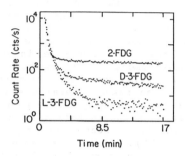

Figure 3. Representative time courses of F-18 in isolated
perfused rat hearts following bolus injection of
fluorosugars. Reproduced with permission from Ref. 49.
Copyright 1984 American Physiological Society.

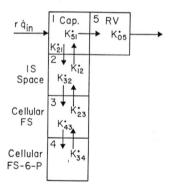

Figure 4. Schematic compartmental model of the rat heart,
showing input of 2FDG (rq_{in}) to the coronary capillaries
(cap.) and its ultimate output from the right ventricle
(RV); IS, interstitium; FS, fluorosugar; FS-6-P,
fluorosugar-6-phosphate; k_{ij}, rate constants for transfer
between compartments.

chemical forms, 2FDG and 2FDG-6-phosphate, and that the only processes going on are transfer of free 2FDG in both directions between capillary and cell, and between cellular free 2FDG and cellular phosphorylated 2FDG. If 2FDG were converted at a significant rate into other chemical forms than the 6-phosphate, then the model might have to be changed or abandoned. Chromatographic analyses of isolated perfused hearts perfused with 2FDG have failed to reveal compounds other than sugar and sugar 6-phosphate. Similar studies with 3FDG, on the other hand revealed two extra peaks (Figure 6), which are probably not present to a sufficient extent to invalidate the model for this sugar. Work with isolated rabbit heart septa has also failed to demonstrate unexpected metabolites of F-18 2FDG (61). However, in vivo NMR studies of the brains of rats infused with high concentrations of F-19 2FDG have indicated formation of metabolites other than the 6-phosphate (62). Whether the difference is due to the organ or the non-tracer methodology (nearly toxic amounts of 2FDG were used in the NMR studies) is not yet clear. The original rationale of this work with isolated hearts was to develop a test bench for PET tracers and protocols. However, our procedures are useful in their own right for investigating fundamental questions of metabolic regulation. For example, Table II gives provisional estimates of interstitial and cellular equilibrium distribution volumes for 2FDG, and of the fractions of administered 2FDG which are transported into the cell and phosphorylated. The values are the mean ± standard deviation for 3 or 4 hearts, except at 2mM perfusate glucose, where we have only succeeded once in maintaining a steady state for the duration of the experiment. The cellular concentration of the glucose analog falls as the perfusate glucose rises, because of competition at the carriers; however, there is no change in the concentration of 2FDG in the interstitium. This confirms that carriers are not involved in transfer of hexoses across the capillary membrane in heart.

Table II. Distribution volumes and transported and phosphorylation fractions for 2FDG

Pre/After load(mmHg)	Perf. glc.(mM)	Vd Int.	Vd Cell	Tranfrac.	Phosfrac.
15/140	2	0.76	0.72	0.056	0.045
15/140	5	0.74±0.10	0.61±019	0.027±0.003	0.020±0.003
15/140	10	0.63±0.14	0.23±0.05	0.012±0.004	0.007±0.002
15/140	15	0.55±0.16	0.37±0.20	0.012±0.003	0.008±0.002
15/140	30	0.65±0.09	0.17±0.03	0.008±0.003	0.003±0.001
5/70	5	0.46±0.10	0.20±0.05	0.010±0.002	0.010±0.002

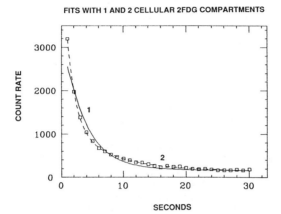

Figure 5. Isolated rat heart data (squares) fitted to the compartmental model of Figure 4 (dotted) and to a simplified model (solid).

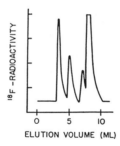

Figure 6. High performance liquid chromatogram if F-18 in rat heart rate after injection of 3-deoxy-3-fluoro-D-glucose. Stationary phase, anion-exchange bonded silica; mobile phase, 20nM potassium phosphate, PH 4.5 Peak assignments in order of elution: 3FDG, unknown, unknown, 3FDG-6-phosphate. (Reproduced with permission from Ref. 49. Copyright 1984 American Physiological Society.)

In addition to calculating biochemical fluxes and concentrations for the glucose analog, we can use residue curve data to infer the cellular content of glucose itself, from the behavior of k^*_{43}, and the independently measured steady-state of glucose metabolism, MRglc. Since MRglc equals the intracellular glucose pool size times k_{43}, we can calculate the metabolic rate with k^*_{43} provided that we know the relationship between k_{43} and k^*_{43}. It can easily be shown that k^*_{43}/k_{43} is constant and independent of the sugar concentration, and that

$$k^*_{43}/k_{43} = V^*max/K^*m \times Km/Vmax \qquad (1)$$

where Km and Vmax are the Michaelis-Menton parameters for hexokinase. Literature data for yeast hexokinase indicate a value of k^*_{43}/k_{43} close to 0.5. We can calculate a value for the heart by considering the term LC (for lumped constant, see e.g. (10)) which relates the metabolic rates (MR) of fluorosugar and glucose at unit plasma concentration.

$$LC = MR_{2FDG}/MR_{glc} \qquad (2)$$

$$= V_{2FDG} \times k^*_{43}/V_{glc} \times k_{43} \qquad (3)$$

where V_{2FDG} and V_{glc} are the ratios of cellular to plasma sugars, and are given by:

$$V_{2FDG} = k^*_{32}/(k^*_{23} + k^*_{43}) \qquad (4)$$

$$V_{glc} = k_{32}/(k_{23} + k_{43}) \qquad (5)$$

When the flux through hexokinase is low relative to the cellular transport step, e.g. at high perfusate glucose concentration, or in the presence of insulin, and $k_{23} > k_{43}$, the equations approximate to $V=k_{32}/k_{23}$. There is good reason to believe that k_{32}/k_{23}, the volume of distribution in the absence of metabolism, has the same value for all sugars sharing the same carrier (59). It follows that when cell transport is rapid compared with phosphorylation

$$LC \text{ (limiting)} = k^*_{43}/k_{43} \qquad (6)$$

A large number of experiments has given the value of 0.56 as the limiting lower bound for LC for 2FDG in the rat heart (64), in good agreement with k^*_{43}/ k_{43} calculated from the hexokinase kinetic parameters (50).

Table III: Preliminary estimates of heart cellular glucose content

Pre/After load (mmHg)	Perfusate glucose (mM)	MRglc (mmol/min/g)	Cellular glucose content (micromol/heart)	Lumped constant
15/140	2	9.7	1.95	0.52
15/140	5	11.6±1.0	2.10±.36	1.19±.39
15/140	10	12.1±1.7	1.71±.40	1.70±.51
15/140	15	11.4±1.6	1.59±.14	1.59±.20
15/140	30	12.2±2.5	1.59±.27	2.39±.40
5/70	5	4.6±0.6	1.18±.31	0.72±.09

Table III gives estimates of the glucose content for the same groups of hearts as Table II. Our data show that cellular glucose content rises with perfusate glucose, but less than linearly. In other words, transport is saturable. Under low workload conditions, where the rate of glucose utilization was about half that at high workloads, glucose content was decreased. This suggests modulation of the transport step by metabolic needs.

Table III also gives values for the lumped constant, which tends to decrease with higher perfusate glucose. Preliminary studies have been done in hearts treated with metabolic inhibitors, in hearts perfused with long chain fatty acids in addition to glucose, and in hearts treated with insulin. In the latter situation there is a large decrease in lumped constant and a rise in estimated cellular glucose content. Insulin is well known to stimulate glucose transport in heart, probably by increasing the number of active carriers (65), but it also has several other effects. The fall in lumped constant to 0.56 reflects the change in relative control strengths (66) of transport and phosphorylation in the presence and absence of insulin. With the hormone, the control strength of transport is very small, and the lumped constant reflects almost purely the relative activities of 2FDG and glucose with hexokinase. The analog is phosphorylated more slowly than the mother substance. The value of the lumped constant under these conditions is more similar to that obtained in normal rat brain (e.g. 10), where there is also a large excess of transport capability over hexokinase activity. Furthermore, isolated yeast hexokinase has an activity ratio (Vmax/Km) for 2FDG half that of glucose (50). When the control strength of transport is high, in hearts perfused without insulin, the lumped constant reflects primarily the relative activities of 2FDG and glucose for the carrier. The analog is the better substrate for transport, and thus the lumped constant rises.

PET Studies

The extensive use of 2FDG in human positron emission tomographic studies is assured. Its vast potential in clinical and experimental work has driven the development of its synthesis to high yield and purity, and will assure its availability for both PET and non-PET applications in the future. It is beyond the scope of this chapter to discuss PET studies of local values of the rate of glucose utilization generated with 2FDG. However, it may be worth pointing out that small volumes in the quantitative images generated by PET scanners can be regarded somewhat like an isolated perfused organ; the isolation is tomographic, rather than physical. Figure 7 shows tomographic data from a human brain gray matter region obtained with 3FDG (51). Two computer generated fits are shown. The two parameters referred to in the lower panel are rate constants for transfer of 3FDG between capillary blood and the pool of free 3FDG in brain. The fit in the upper panel also takes into account rate constants for phosphorylation and dephosphorylation, analogous to k^*_{43} and k^*_{34} in Figure 4. The best estimates of the transport rate constant are obtained when corrections for the slow phosphorylation of 3FDG are made. Thus, the transport of 3FDG through the blood brain barrier can be studied in small regions of the human brain. Corresponding estimates made with 2FDG are more uncertain because the correction for phosphorylation is much greater.

Conclusions

We have shown that individual rate constants in residue curves obtained with isolated perfused rat hearts can be measured with much greater precision than the corresponding parameters in PET. A single study with 2FDG yields good values of cell membrane extraction, dephosphorylation rate constant and fluorosugar distribution volume in addition to the fluorosugar phosphorylation rate. From a series of 2FDG studies and an independent measure of the rate of glucose utilization, the glucose content of the hearts can be calculated under a range of conditions.

After spending six years developing our approach, we now plan to extend it to studies of hearts under abnormal metabolic conditions, such as ischemia and hypoxia. We will also be able to examine the effects of hormones and of pharmacologically active compounds in a novel way. We also expect the use of F-18 labeled fluorosugars in isolated perfused organs to continue its interactive relationship with PET. On the one hand, new tracers and administration protocols can be explored much more quickly and cheaply than in imaging studies. On the other, it may be possible to attack questions generated by patient studies, such as those relating to changes in the value of the lumped constant in pathological conditions.

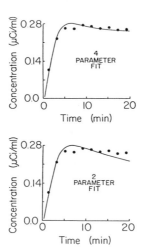

Figure 7. Time course of F-18 in human brain after intravenous injection of 3FDG. Upper panel, fit allowing for metabolism to a tapped species such as 3FDG-6-phosphate; lower panel, fit assuming no metabolism.

Acknowledgments

This work was funded by the National Institutes of Health under Grants HL29046, HL27970 and HL36534.

Literature Cited

1. Phelps M.E.; Mazziota J.; Schelbert H. Positron Emission Tomography and Quantitative Autoradiography; Raven Press: New York, 1986.
2. Palmer A.J.; Taylor D.M. (Eds): Radiopharmaceuticals Labeled with Halogen Isotopes. Published as Int. J. Appl.Radiat. Isotopes 37, 645-921, 1986.
3. Lederer C.M.; Shirley V.M. (Eds) Table of Isotopes. (7th edition); Wiley: New York, 1978.
4. Nickles, R.J.; Gatley, S.J.; Votaw, J.R.; Kornguth, M.L. Int. J. Appl. Radiat. Isotopes 1986, 37, 649-661.
5. Reivich M.; Kuhl D.; Wolf A.P.; Greenberg J.; Phelps M.; Ido T.; Casella V.; Hoffman E.; Alavi A.; Sokoloff L. Circulation Res. 1979, 44, 127-137.
6. Sokoloff L. Thr Harvey Lectures. Series 79, 1985, pp 77-143.
7. Sols A.; Crane R.A. J. Biol. Chem 1954, 210, 581-595.
8. Gallagher B.M.; Ansari A.; Atkins H.; Casella V.; Christman D.R.; Fowler J.S.; Ido T.; MacGregor R.R.; Som P.; Wan C-N.; Wolf A.P.; Kuhl D.E.; Reivich M. J. Nucl. Med. 1977, 18, 990-996.
9. Gjedde A.; Wienhard K.; Heiss W-D.; Kloster G.; Diemer N.H.; Herholz K.; Pawlik G. J. Cereb. Blood Flow Metab. 1985, 5, 163-178.
10. Sokoloff, L.; Reivich, M.; Kennedy, C.; DesRosiers, M.; Patlak, C.S.; Pettigrew, K.D.; Sakarada, O.; Shinohara, M. J. Neurochem. 1977, 28, 897-916.
11. Reivich M.; Alavi A.; Wolf A.; Fowler J.; Russell J.; Arnett D.; MacGregor R.R.; Shiue C-Y.; Atkins H.; Anand A.; Dann R.; Greenberg J.H. J. Cereb .Blood Flow Metab. 1985, 5, 179-192.
12. Fowler J.S.; Finn R.D.; Lambrecht R.M.; Wolf A.P. J. Nucl. Med. 1973, 14, 63-64.
13. Nickles R.J.; Daube M.E. Int. J. Appl. Radiat. Isot. 1984, 35, 117-122.
14. Bida G.T.; Satyamurthy N.; Barrio J.R. J. Nucl. Med. 1984, 25, 1327-1334.
15. Schrobilgen G.; Firnau G.; Chirakal R.; Garnett E.S. J. Chem. Soc. Chem. Commun. 1981, 198-199.
16. Chirakal R.; Firnau G.; Schrobilgen G.J.; McKay J.; Garnett E.S. Int. J. Appl. Radiat. Isot. 1984, 35, 401-404.
17. Palmer A.J.; Clark J.C.; Goulding R.W. Int.J.Appl.Radiat. Isot. 1977, 28, 53-65.
18. DeKleijn J.P. J. Fluorine Chem. 1977, 10, 341-350.
19. Landini, D., Maia, A.; and Podda, G. J. Org. Chem. 1982, 47, 2264-2268.
20. Gatley S.J.; Shaughnessy W.J. J. Labelled. Compounds 1981, 18, 24-25.
21. Gatley S.J.; Kornguth M.L.; De Grado T.R.; Holden J.E. J. Nucl. Med. 1987, 28, 635.
22. Rosenthal, M.S.; Bosch, A.L.; Nickles, R.J.; Gatley, S.J. Int. J. Appl. Radiat. Isotopes 1985, 36, 318.

23. Fowler, J.S.; Wolf, A.P. Int. J. Appl. Radiat. Isotopes 1986, 37, 663-668.
24. Ido T.; Wan C-N.; Fowler J.S.; Wolf A.P. J. Org. Chem. 1977, 42, 2341-2342.
25. Shiue C-Y.; Salvadori P.A.; Wolf A.P.; Fowler J.S.; MacGregor R.R. J. Nucl. Med. 1982, 23, 899-903.
26. Adam M.J. J. Chem. Soc. Chem. Commun. 1982, 730-731.
27. Jewett D.M.; Potocki J.F.; Ehrenkaufer R.E. J. Fluorine Chem. 1984, 24, 477-484.
28. Ehrenkaufer R.E.; Potocki J.F.; Jewett D.M. J. Nucl. Med. 1984, 25, 333-337.
29. Shiue C-Y.; Fowler J.S.; Wolf A.P.; Alexoff D.; MacGregor R.R. J. Labelled Compd. Radiopharm. 1985, 22, 503.
30. Shiue C-Y.; To K.C.; Wolf A.P. J. Labelled Compd. Radiopharm 1983, 20, 157.
31. Sood S.; Firnau G.; Garnett ES. Int. J. Appl. Radiat. Isot. 1983, 34, 743-745.
32. Shaughnessy W.J.; Gatley S.J.; Hichwa R.D.; Lieberman L.M.; Nickles R.J. Int. J. Appl. Radiat. Isotopes 1981, 32, 23-29.
33. Casella V.; Ido T.; Wolf A.P.; Fowler J.S.; MacGregor R.R.; Ruth T.J. J. Nucl. Med. 1980, 21, 750-757.
34. Bida G.T.; Ehrenkaufer R.L.; Wolf A.P.; Fowler J.S.; MacGregor R.R.; Ruth T.J. J. Nucl. Med. 1980, 21, 758-762.
35. Tewson T.J. J. Nucl. Med. 1983, 24, 718-721.
36. Tewson T.J. J. Org. Chem. 1983, 48, 3507.
37. Hutchins L.G.; Bosch A.L.; Rosenthal M.S.; Nickles R.J.; Gatley S.J. Int. J. Appl. Radiat. Isot 1985, 36, 375-378.
38. Tewson T.J.; Soderlind M. J. Nucl. Med. 1985, 26, 129.
39. Levy S.; Livine E.; Elmaleh D.; Curatolo W. J. Chem. Soc. Chem. Commun. 1982, 972-973.
40. Haradahira, T.; Maeda, M.; Omae, H.; Kojima, M. J. Label. Compd. Radiopharm. 1984, 21, 1218-1219.
41. Hamacher, K.; Coenen, H.H.; Stocklin, G. J. Nucl. Med. 1986, 27, 235-238.
42. Beeley P.A.; Szarek W.A.; Hay G.W.; Perlmutter M.M. Can. J. Chem 1984, 62, 2709-2711.
43. Christman D.R.; Ohranovic Z.; Shreave W.W. J. Labeled Compd. Radiopharm. 1977, 13, 555-559.
44. Tewson T.J.; Welch M.J. J. Org. Chem. 1978, 43, 1090-1099.
45. Tewson T.J.; Welch M.J.; Raichle M.E. J. Nucl. Med. 1978, 19, 1339-1345.
46. Shaughnessy W.J.; Gatley S.J. Int. J. Appl. Radiat. Isot. 1980, 31, 339-341.
47. Foster, A.B.; Hems, R.; Webber, J.M. Carbohyd. Res. 1967, 5, 292-301.
48. Goodman, M.M.; Elmaleh, D.R.; Kearfoot, K.J.; Ackerman, R.H.; Hoop, B.; Brownell, G.L.; Alpert, N.M.; Strauss, H.W. J. Nucl. Med. 1981, 22, 138-144.
49. Halama J.R.; Gatley S.J.; DeGrado T.R.; Bernstein D.R.; Ng C.K.; Holden J.E. Am. J. Physiol. 1984, 247, H756-H759.
50. Bessell E.M.; Foster A.B.; Westwood J.H. Biochem. J. 1972, 128, 199-204.
51. Koeppe R.A. Ph.D. Thesis. University of Wisconsin, 1985.
52. Ido, T.; Wan, C-N.; Casella, V.; Fowler, J.S.; Wolf, A.P.; Reivich, M.; Kuhl, D.E. J. Label. Comp. Radiopharm. 1978, 14, 175-18.

53. Haradahira, T.; Maeda, M.; Omae, H.; Yano, Y.; Kojima, M. Chem. Pharm. Bull. 1984, 32, 4758-4766.
54. Luxen, A.; Satyamurthy, N.; Bida, G.T.; Barrio, J.R. Int. J. Appl. Radiat. Isotopes 1986, 37, 409-414.
55. Imahori, Y.; Ido, T.; Ishiwata, K.; Takahashi, T.; Kawashima, K.; Yanai, K.; Miura, Y.; Mouma, M.; Watanabe, S.; and Ujiie, A. Annual Report of the Cyclotron and Radioisotope Center, Tohoku University, 1984, pp 119-130.
56. Gatley S.J.; Martin J.A.; Cooper M.D. J. Nucl. Med. 1987, 28, 624.
57. Gatley, S.J.; Shaughnessy, W.J. Int. J. Appl. Radiat. Isotopes 1982, 33, 1325-1330.
58. Nickles, R.J.; Hutchins, G.D.; Daube, M.E. J. Nucl. Med. 1982, 23, p60.
59. Taegtmeyer, H.; Hems, R.; Krebs, H.A. Biochem. J. 1980, 186, 701-711.
60. Chu, S.C.; Berman, M. Communications of the ACM 1974, 17, 699-702.
61. Halama J.R. Ph.D. Thesis. University of Wisconsin, 1983.
62. Krivokapich, J.; Huang, S.C.; Phelps, M.E.; Barrio, J.R.; Watanabe, C.R.; Selin, E.E.; Shine, K.I. Am. J. Physiol. 1982, 243, H884-H896.
63. Nakada, T.; Kwee, I.L.; Conboy, C.B. J. Neurochem. 1986, 46, 198.
64. Ng, C.K.; Holden, J.E.; DeGrado, T.R.; Kornguth, M.L.; Raffel, D.M.; Gatley, S.J. J. Nucl. Med. 1986, 27, 966.
65. Cheung, J.Y.; Conover, C.; Regen, D.M.; Whitfield, C.F.; Morgan, H.E. Am. J. Physiol. 1978, 234, E70-E78.
66. Kacser, H.; Burns, J.A. Biochem. Soc. Trans. 1979, 7, 1149-1160.

RECEIVED February 5, 1988

Chapter 10

Antiviral Activities of 2'-Fluorinated Arabinosyl–Pyrimidine Nucleosides

J. J. Fox[1], K. A. Watanabe[1], T. C. Chou[1], R. F. Schinazi[2], K. F. Soike[3], I. Fourel[4], G. Hantz[4], and C. Trepo[4]

[1]Memorial Sloan–Kettering Cancer Center, New York, NY 10021
[2]Emory University–Veterans Administration Medical Center, Atlanta, GA 30033
[3]Delta Regional Primate Research Center, Covington, LA 70433
[4]Hepatitis Virus Unit, Institut National de la Santé et de la Recherche Médicale, U 271, 69003 Lyon, France

Comparative biochemical and antiviral studies are described for the 2'-fluoro-substituted arabinosyl-pyrimidine nucleosides 1-(2'-deoxy-2'-fluoro-β-D-arabinofuranosyl)-5-methyluracil [FMAU] and 1-(2'-deoxy-2'-fluoro-β-D-arabinofuranosyl)-5-ethyluracil [FEAU]. Biochemical studies indicated that FEAU should be a selective antiherpesvirus agent that is less toxic than FMAU. FEAU was evaluated against simian varicella virus infection in African green monkeys and, like FMAU, was highly effective in preventing rash and reducing viremia without apparent toxicity at doses of 30, 10, or 3 mg/kg/day x 10 administered intravenously. Oral administration of FEAU in those monkeys at 10, 3, and 1 mg/kg/day x 10 was equally effective.

FEAU and FMAU were evaluated against woodchuck hepatitis virus (WHV) in chronically-infected wood-chucks (an animal model of choice for evaluation of potential antihepatitis B virus agents in humans). FEAU inhibits WHV replication at 2.0 and 0.2 mg/kg/day x 10 in all animals tested. The inhibitory effect was immediate, nontoxic and long-lasting. Preliminary studies indicated that FEAU is also effective against WHV when given by the oral route. FMAU also produced immediate inhibitory effects against WHV replication at doses of 2.0 and 0.2 mg/kg/day x 5; however, unacceptable toxicities were observed with FMAU at these dosages.

FEAU appears to be the most promising of the nucleoside analogs tested thus far against Hepadna-viridae and may be an effective agent clinically against Hepatitis B virus.

0097–6156/88/0374–0176$06.00/0

Since our original report (1) on the synthesis and anti-herpes virus
activities of several 5-substituted pyrimidine nucleosides bearing
the 1-(2'-deoxy-2'-fluoro-β-D-arabinofuranosyl) moiety, structure-
activity studies have indicated that the 2'-fluoro substituent in the
"up" (arabino) configuration conferred more potent antiviral
activity than did a 2'-OH, hydrogen, or other halogens (2).
Moreover, where studied (3,4), the 2'-fluoro nucleosides were
resistant to catabolic cleavage by nucleoside phosphorylases,
presumably a result of the increased metabolic stability of the N-
glycosyl linkage imposed by this electronegative 2'-substituent. Of
the several 2'-fluoro-5-substituted-arabinosyl pyrimidine nucleosides
synthesized (1), 1-(2'-deoxy-2'-fluoro-β-D-arabinofuranosyl)-5-iodo-
cytosine [FIAC] has demonstrated clinical efficacy against Herpes-
virus infections in Phase 1 (5) and against Varicella zoster virus in
Phase 2 (6) clinical trials in immunocompromised cancer patients.
The corresponding 5-methyluracil analog, 1-(2'-deoxy-2'-fluoro-β-D-
arabinofuranosyl)-5-methyluracil [FMAU] was found to be more potent
in mice infected with Herpes simplex virus (HSV) types 1 and 2
without toxicity at effective dose levels. FMAU was also found to be
active in vitro and in vivo against P-815 and L-1210 leukemia cell
lines resistant to the antileukemic agent, 1-β-D-arabinofuranosyl-
cytosine [Ara-C]. A Phase 1 trial of FMAU in patients with advanced
cancer showed that drug-induced central nervous system (CNS) dys-
function was the dose-limiting toxicity (7).

FIAC   FMAU   FEAU

With FMAU as a lead compound, the syntheses of other 5-alkyl
substituted 2'-fluoro-ara-uracils were undertaken (8,9) including 1-
(2'-deoxy-2'-fluoro-β-D-arabinofuranosyl)-5-ethyluracil [FEAU]. As
shown in Table I, though FEAU was approximately one log order less
potent than FMAU against HSV-1 and HSV-2 infected Vero cells in
culture, the former exhibited far less host cell toxicity, resulting
in an extremely favorable therapeutic index (9,10).
    A comparison of the antiviral activity of FMAU, FEAU, and 5-
ethyl-2'-deoxyuridine (EDU) in mice inoculated intracerebrally with
HSV-2 is given in Table II (10). FEAU showed activity at 50
mg/kg/day for 4 days and was highly effective in reducing mortality
in these mice at doses of 100 - 200 mg/kg/day. At these dose levels,
no toxicity was observed. In normal (uninfected) mice, FEAU

Table I. Comparative Anti-HSV Activity of FMAU and FEAU in
Plaque Reduction Assays in Vero Cells

	HSV-1(F)*		HSV-2(G)*		ID_{50}#	Therapeutic Index	
	ED_{50}** (μM)	ED_{90}	ED_{50} (μM)	ED_{90}	(μM)	ID_{50}/ED_{90} HSV-1	HSV-2
FMAU	0.010	0.042	0.023	0.09	2.8	67	31
FEAU	0.024	0.26	0.24	0.91	>200	>769	>220

*Correlation coefficient $\geq$ 0.86. #Cytotoxic effect measured in
rapidly dividing cells. ID_{50} = concentration required to inhibit
cell growth by 50%. **ED = Effective dose required to inhibit
HSV replication by the percentage indicated.

Table II. Antiviral Effects of FEAU, FMAU and EDU in Mice Inoculated
Intracerebrally with HSV-2 (Strain G)

Treatment	Dose* mg/kg/day	MDD**	% Survivors	%Wt Gain on Day§ 7	14	21	30
Neg Control (no virus)	–		100	–3	9	13	16
PBSΔ (virus control)	6.7		7	–22	–14[+]	8[+]	17[+]
FEAU	10	9.4	8	–7	–13[+]	31[+]	36[+]
	50	11.8	25	3	–10	16	25
	100	11.0	72	2	7	13	13
	200	(14)#	93	0	1	9	13
FMAU	0.5	9.4	67	1	4	5	7
EDU	800	7.6	13	–10	–6	2	6
	1000	8.6	33	3	13	34	43

*Given 5 hr after intracerebral inoculation. Dose schedule, twice a
day for 4 days. **Median day of death calculated on day 21.
#Numbers in parentheses indicate death of a single animal. §As
compared to day 1. [+]Based on weight of a single surviving animal
only. ΔPhosphate buffer saline.

was nontoxic at doses of 800 mg/kg/day given twice daily for four
days. It is also noteworthy that EDU, which differs structurally
from FEAU only by the absence of the 2'-fluoro substituent, is much
less effective than FEAU in this HSV-2 mouse encephalitis model.
This finding is consistent with our previous observation (1)
attesting to the importance of the 2'-fluoro substituent for the
anti-HSV activity exhibited by these arabinofuranosyl-pyrimidine
nucleosides.

It was concluded previously (11) that FMAU is a most potent and
selective antiviral compound for the treatment of mouse encephalitis
caused by HSV-2 and therefore deserved consideration as a potential
agent in human trials for the treatment of HSV encephalitis in
neonates and adults at low dose levels. The preliminary data
described in Tables I and II for FEAU suggested (10) that this
compound may also be worthy of similar consideration. Based upon
these earlier findings (10) and on our preliminary biochemical report
(12), further comparative biochemical and antiviral studies were
undertaken with FMAU and FEAU, including their relative activities
against Simian varicella virus in the African green monkey and
against hepatitis virus in the woodchuck animal model. In these
studies (13) an alternative synthesis of FEAU is also described.

COMPARATIVE BIOCHEMICAL STUDIES

Biochemical studies at Memorial Sloan-Kettering Cancer Center (13) on
the relative effects of FEAU and FMAU on the growth of mammalian
cells is shown in Table III. Note that against the human

Table III. Comparison of Effects of FEAU and FMAU in Mammalian Cells*

ED_{50} (in μM) for Inhibiting Cell growth in:	FEAU	FMAU	FEAU/FMAU
HL-60 Cells	2060	15.4	133
Vero Cells	>200	2.8	>71

ED_{50} (μM) for inhibiting thymidine incorporation into DNA	FEAU	FMAU	FEAU/FMAU
P-815 Cells	700	14.0	50
L-1210 Cells	630	28.0	22
Rat Bone Marrow Cells	3,700	8.9	415

*See reference 13 for experimental procedures

promyelocytic leukemia cell line (HL-60) as well as against Vero
cells (derived from the African green monkey), FEAU is far less
growth-inhibitory than FMAU, which compares favorably to the in vitro
study given in Table I. Similarly, against rodent cell lines (P-815,
L-1210 and rat bone marrow cells), FEAU is substantially less
inhibitory of thymidine incorporation than FMAU (Table III).

Cellular kinetic constants (K_i) were also determined (13) for the inhibition of natural precursor incorporation into the DNA of L-1210 cells by FEAU and FMAU. Using tritium-labelled natural precursors as substrates (thymidine, 2'-deoxyuridine and 2'-deoxycytidine), it was found that the FEAU/FMAU K_i ratios were 61, 111, and 8.1, respectively. These results also indicated that FEAU is a weaker inhibitor of natural nucleoside anabolism than FMAU in these mammalian cells.

Table IV.   Incorporation of [2-^{14}C] FEAU or [2-^{14}C]FMAU
Into DNA of Mammalian Cells

Incorporation at 10 μM (in p mole/10^6 cells/hr)

Cell Line	FEAU	FMAU
L-1210	ND*	0.69
Vero	ND*	1.3
HSV-1 Infected Vero Cells	0.48	3.4

*Not detectable.   Also not detectable at 100 μM.

Studies on the incorporation of 2-^{14}C-labelled FEAU and FMAU into the DNA of mammalian cells showed very significant differences (Table IV). There was no detectable incorporation of FEAU radioactivity into the DNA of either L-1210 or Vero cell lines, but substantial amounts of FMAU radioactivity were incorporated into the DNA of both cell lines. When HSV-1 infected Vero cells were exposed to ^{14}C-labelled FEAU and FMAU, both nucleosides were incorporated into the DNA of these virus-infected cells. Under these conditions, FMAU incorporation into HSV-1 infected Vero cells was 7-fold greater than that observed for FEAU. This difference in incorporation may be due to the greater affinity of FMAU for viral-encoded DNA polymerase and is comparable to the magnitude of the difference of their anti-herpetic potencies in vitro (13).

It is generally accepted that the selective antiherpes activity of 2'-fluoro-arabinosylpyrimidine nucleosides is associated in large measure with their ability to be recognized as good substrates for HSV-specified thymidine kinase (TK), but not by the host TK (14,15). As shown in Table V, FMAU is a good substrate (relative to thymidine) for cytosol and mitochondrial TK's derived from the HL-60 human cell line, as well as for HSV-1 and HSV-2 derived TK's. By contrast, FEAU is a very poor substrate for the host HL-60 derived cytosol TK and an excellent substrate for HSV-1 and HSV-2 derived TK's (13). These data are consistent with the recent report by Mansuri et al., (16) who showed that FEAU has a very low affinity for Vero cell TK (compared to thymidine) but a high affinity toward HSV-1 and HSV-2 encoded TK's. Their data also indicate that, in uninfected Vero cells, FEAU would be phosphorylated at a very low rate in the presence of thymidine. Their report (16) also describes a modified chemical synthesis of FEAU.

Table V. Percentage Rates of Phosphorylation of FEAU and FMAU
(Relative to Thymidine*) by Various Thymidine Kinases**

Enzyme Source	% Rates of Phosphorylation of Various Thymidine Kinases	
	FEAU	FMAU
HL-60 Cells		
Cytosol TK	0 - 2.1	81.7
Mitochondrial TK	N/A#	219.0
HSV-1 (Strain KOS) TK	82.7	42.0
HSV-2 (Strain 333) TK	203.2	146.6

*Thymidine at 400 μM. **Measured by procedure of Cheng,
et al., (14). #Not assayed.

These biochemical and antiviral screening studies
(10,12-16) suggest that FEAU should be more selective in its
antiviral activity and thus offer less host toxicity. In vivo
experiments in mice (10,13) show that both FMAU and FEAU are
relatively nontoxic. However, FMAU is very neurotoxic in dogs
(lethal dose 2.5 mg/kg/day, i.v. x 5), while preliminary studies on
FEAU in dogs at 50 mg/kg/day x 10 show no encephalopathy (lethal dose
100 mg/kg/day x 10). As mentioned previously, FMAU exhibited dose-
limiting CNS toxicity in patients with advanced cancer (7) at an
intravenous dose of 0.8 mg/kg/day x 5. The toxicity of FEAU in
humans is not known.

COMPARATIVE STUDIES IN MONKEYS AGAINST SIMIAN VARICELLA VIRUS.

Studies at the Delta Regional Primate Research Center compared the
activities of FEAU and FMAU in African green monkeys infected with
simian varicella virus (SVV). As shown in Table VI, the three
untreated controls exhibited marked viremia and died by day 11.
Monkeys treated with FEAU at three dose levels (intravenous route)
showed no apparent toxicity even at the higher dose of 30 mg/kg/day x
10. Hematology tests and serum chemistries for all treated monkeys
were normal and viremia (relative to the controls) was minimal even
at the low dose of 3 mg/kg/day. While the control monkeys developed
severe rash, none of the FEAU-treated monkeys developed rash at these
drug levels. Further studies showed that a lower dose of 1 mg/kg/day
prevented development of rash but did not reduce viremia in two out
of three monkeys. These data suggest that the minimal effective dose
in this system for FEAU is ~1 mg/kg/day. Concurrent studies with
FMAU showed it to be ~40-fold more potent against SVV with a minimal
effective dose of ~0.04 mg/kg/day x 10.
FEAU was also highly effective in the treatment of Simian
varicella virus by the oral route. Oral administration at dose
levels of 10, 3, or 1 mg/kg/day x 10 prevented rash (Table VII) and
reduced viremia significantly. Even at the 1 mg dose, rash was
almost entirely prevented (two vesicles appeared on day 9, then
promptly disappeared). Doses at 10 mg/kg/day x 10 by the oral route

Table VI. Evaluation of FEAU in Treatment of Simian Varicella Virus
Infection in the African Green Monkey: Effect on Viremia

Treatment Group*	Monkey Number	Viremia** – Mean PFU on Days p.i.				
		3	5	7	9	11
Control – H$_2$O	G029	1	140	>400	Dead	
	G030	3	163	>400	>400	Dead
	G031	1	99	>400	Dead	
FEAU – 30 mg/kg/day	G023	1	0	0	0	0
	G024	2	0	0	0	0
FEAU – 10 mg/kg/day	G025	1	14	5	0	0
	G026	0	1	1	0	0
FEAU – 3 mg/kg/day	G027	1	8	0	0	0
	G028	0	1	1	0	0

*Treatment was administered by i.v. injection twice daily beginning
48 hours after virus inoculation and continuing for ten days
**Viremia was determined by culture of lymphocytes collected from
3 mL of heparinized blood on indicated days post-infection (p.i.).
The mean plaque-forming units expressed is the average number of
plaques present in two flasks of Vero cell co-cultures inoculated
with each lymphocyte suspension.

were without any observed toxicity. Thus, FEAU is shown to be a
highly effective and selective antiviral in the treatment of SVV
infection by both the intravenous and oral routes.
     In view of: a) the in vitro activity (15,18) of FIAC and FMAU
against varicella zoster virus (VZV, a member of the human herpes-
virus group), b) the reported efficacy of FIAC for the treatment of
varicella zoster virus in Phase 2 trials in immunosuppressed patients
(6), and c) the in vivo activities of FMAU and FEAU against simian
varicella virus described herein and elsewhere (18), one may expect
that FEAU will also exhibit significant selective activity against
VZV in humans.

COMPARATIVE ANTI-HEPATITIS VIRUS STUDIES IN WOODCHUCKS.

Hepatitis B virus (HBV), a member of the Hepadna viruses, causes
acute and chronic hepatitis in humans. It is estimated that ~200
million people are carriers of this virus. HBV may be the primary
causative agent of hepatocellular carcinoma (19). Hepadna viruses
have also been discovered in other animals such as the woodchuck
(Marmota Monax). The close structural and clinical pathological
similarities, including nucleic acid homology (20), noted between
woodchuck hepatitis virus (WHV) and HBV suggest that the woodchuck
may represent a promising model for studying persistent hepatitis
virus infections as well as their relationship to the development of
liver cancer (21). Like HBV, the woodchuck hepatitis virus

elaborates a very similar DNA polymerase for its replication and integration. Potential anti–HBV agents can be detected by their inhibition of endogenous WHV or HBV DNA polymerase obtained from sera prepared from chronic–carrier woodchucks and from an immunosuppressed patient positive for the hepatitis B surface antigen. Such studies were undertaken at the Hepatitis Virus Unit, INSERM, Lyon, France, to measure the inhibitory effects of certain nucleoside triphosphates on these endogenous viral DNA polymerases.

In a series of assays (23,24, and C. Trepo, personal communication), the relative sensitivities of HBV and WHV DNA polymerases to several nucleoside triphosphates were determined (Table VIII). Of the six nucleoside triphosphates examined, FMAU was the most efficient inhibitor of both HBV and WHV DNA polymerases, followed closely by FIAC. Moreover, the potencies ($ID_{50's}$) of each of these six triphosphates against HBV or WHV DNA polymerases, though not identical, were rather close. More important, the orders of potency as inhibitors of these viral DNA polymerases were identical. These results attest further to the striking similarities between HBV and WHV and point to the validity of the woodchuck as an animal model of choice for the in vivo evaluation of potential antihepatitis B virus agents (24,).

Studies were then undertaken to evaluate FMAU and FEAU in this animal model using woodchucks naturally chronically–infected with woodchuck hepatitis virus (25). [It was assumed that these nucleosides would be anabolized to their nucleoside triphosphates within the animal.] WHV replication was measured periodically by the endogenous DNA polymerase activity and by the detection of WHV DNA by the dot–blot hybridization assay. The viral DNA polymerase activities of untreated woodchucks are given in Figure 1. Three different dosages of FMAU and FEAU were investigated. FMAU at 2.0 mg/kg/day x 5, (given intraperitoneally beginning at day 0), produced marked inhibition of WHV replication as shown by the complete suppression of WHV DNA polymerase activity (Figure 2). However, at this dose, severe CNS toxicity was observed, which was eventually lethal. FEAU administered i.p. at 2.0 mg/kg/day x 10 also produced almost immediate suppression of WHV replication and did not exhibit any toxic effects. At 0.2 mg/kg/day, FMAU (given x 5) and FEAU (given x 10) were equally effective in suppressing viral replication (Figure 3). At this dose, FMAU exhibited a less severe and delayed toxicity, whereas FEAU was again nontoxic. Even at doses of 0.04 mg/kg/day x 10, FEAU exerted a somewhat diminished anti–WHV effect. A preliminary study with one woodchuck given FEAU by oral administration at a dose of 0.2 mg/kg/day x 10 gave significant suppression of WHV replication, again without any observed toxicity (Figure 4).

After cessation of drug administration, the inhibitory activity of FEAU at 0.2 or 2.0 mg doses remained significant over a six–week period while returning slowly to pretreatment levels. FEAU inhibition of WHV replication was almost immediate and was markedly more sustained than is the case with other antivirals such as 6–deoxyacyclovir [9-(2-hydroxyethoxymethyl)-2-aminopurine], DHPG [9-(1,3-dihydroxy-2-propoxymethyl)guanine], or Ara–AMP [9-(β-D-

Table VII. Evaluation of Oral Dosage of FEAU in the Treatment of
Simian Varicella Virus Infection in the African Green Monkey:
Effect on Rash[#]

Treatment Group*	Monkey Number	Rash − Severity on Days p.i.							
		6	7	8	9	10	11	12	14
Control − PBS**	F644	±	3+	4+	4+	Dead			
	G668	−	−	±	2+	1+	±	±	−
	G604	−	±	3+	4+	4+	2+	+	+
FEAU − 10 mg/kg/day	G249	−	−	−·	−	−	−	−	−
	G267	−	−	−	−	−	−	−	−
	G264	−	−	−	−	−	−	−	−
FEAU − 3 mg/kg/day	G665	−	−	−	−	−	−	−	−
	G257	−	−	−	−	−	−	−	−
	G268	−	−	−	−	−	−	−	−
FEAU − 1 mg/kg/day	G269	−	−	−	−	−	−	−	−
	G270	−	−	−	−	−	−	−	−
	G274	−	−	−	±	−	−	−	−

*Treatment was administered by stomach tube twice daily beginning 48
hours after virus inoculation and continuing for ten days.
**Phosphate buffer saline. #Severity of rash was graded on a scale
of ± to 4+. A ± rash was scored when several vesicles were observed
while a 4+ rash indicated the widespread distribution of rash over
the body surface.

Table VIII. Comparative Inhibitory Activities of Nucleoside
Triphosphate Analogs on DNA Polymerases of Human Hepatitis Virus
(HBV) and Woodchuck Hepatitis Virus (WHV)

Inhibitors**	ID_{50} (μM)*	
	HBV DNA Polymerase[+]	WHV DNA Polymerase[+]
FMAU−TP	0.025	0.05
FIAC−TP	0.05	0.10
BVDU−TP	0.25	0.30
Ara T−TP	0.30	0.40
ACV−TP	0.90	0.70
Ara C−TP	1.10	1.20

*ID50 = Concentration of inhibitor giving 50% inhibition of DNA
polymerase activity. **These inhibitors are the nucleoside 5'-
triphosphate derivatives of: FMAU, 1-(2'-deoxy-2'-fluoro-β-D-
arabinofuranosyl)-5-methyluracil; FIAC, 1-(2'-deoxy-2'-fluoro-β-D-
arabinofuranosyl)-5-iodocytosine; BVDU, E-5(2-bromovinyl)-2'-
deoxyuridine; Ara-T, 1-β-D-arabinofuranosylthymine; ACV, 9-(2-
hydroxyethoxymethyl)guanine; Ara-A, 9-β-D-arabinofuranosyladenine.
[+]DNA polymerase was assayed as described by Kaplan et al. (22), as
modified by Hantz et al. (23)

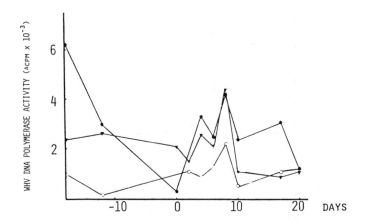

Figure 1.   WHV DNA Polymerase Activity in Untreated Chronically
Infected Woodchucks (Controls).
Each symbol (○—◌, ▼—▼, or ●—●) represents individual woodchucks, with
points on the line indicating the day when blood was taken for
polymerase assay.   DNA polymerase activity was measured as described
by Kaplan et al. (22), as modified by Hantz et al. (23).

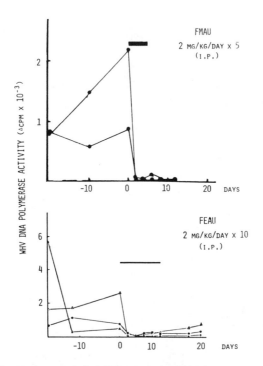

Figure 2. Comparison of Inhibition of WHV Replication in
Chronically infected Woodchucks by Treatment with FMAU and FEAU at
Dosage and Schedule Indicated.
The length of the bar gives the drug treatment time period in days
indicated on the abscissa. Each of the symbols (△—△, ●—●, or ▲—▲)
refers to individual woodchucks, with points on the line representing
the days when bloods were drawn for polymerase assay. WHV DNA
polymerase activity was measured according to Kaplan et al. (22), as
modified by Hantz et al. (23).

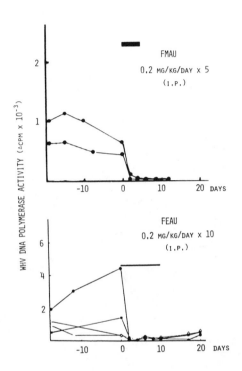

Figure 3. Inhibition of WHV Replication in Chronically Infected Woodchucks by Treatment with FMAU and FEAU at Lower Dosages. (See Figure 2 for legend).

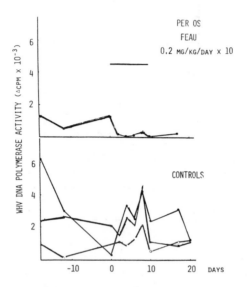

Figure 4. Inhibition of WHV Replication in Chronically Infected Woodchucks Treated with FEAU by the Oral Route. FEAU was administered by stomach tube. (See Figures 1 and 2 for legend.)

arabinofuranosyl)adenine 5'-phosphate. These latter drugs also
diminished WHV DNA polymerase levels, but they soon rebounded to
pretreatment levels after cessation of drug administration (C, Trepo,
personal communication). In contrast to previous results obtained
with FMAU and FIAC (where lethal toxicity was demonstrated), only an
~10% weight loss was observed following FEAU treatment (24).
   The observed efficacy of FEAU against woodchuck hepatitis virus
replication at these low doses was rather surprising. On the basis
of the in vitro studies on Herpes simplex viruses (9,10), the in vivo
studies on the herpes encephalitis model in mice (10), and the simian
varicella virus studies in the African green monkey reported herein,
one would have expected that FEAU would be much less potent than
FMAU. The data suggest that FEAU may be an effective agent
clinically against hepatitis B virus. On the basis of its potency
and selectivity, it appears to be the most promising of the
nucleoside analogs tested thus far. Further evaluation of FEAU is in
progress.

ACKNOWLEDGMENTS

These studies were supported in part by National Cancer Institute
grants CA-08748, 18601 and 18856 (JJF, KAW, TCC), by CA-44094 and The
Veterans Administration (RFS), by the National Institute of Allergy
and Infectious Diseases grant NO-A1-62521 (KFS), and by the Institut
National de la Santé et de Recherche Médicale (IF, OH, CT).

LITERATURE CITED

1. Watanabe, K. A.; Reichman, U.; Hirota, K.; Lopez, C.; Fox, J. J.
    J. Med. Chem. 1979, 22 21-24.
2. Fox, J. J.; Lopez, C.; Watanabe, K. A., in Medicinal Chemistry
    Advances; de las Heras, F. G.; Vega, S., Eds.; Pergamon Press:
    Oxford, 1981; pp 27-40.
3. Chou, T. C.; Feinberg, A.; Grant, A. J.; Vidal, P.; Reichman, U.;
    Watanabe, K. A.; Fox, J. J. Cancer Res. 1981, 41, 3336-3342.
4. Coderre, J. A.; Santi, D. V.; Matsuda, A.; Watanabe, K. A.;
    Fox, J. J. J. Med. Chem. 1983, 26, 1149-1152.
5. Young, C. W.; Schneider, R.; Leyland-Jones, B.; Armstrong, D.;
    Tan, C.; Lopez, C.; Watanabe, K. A.; Fox, J. J.; Philips, F. S.
    Cancer Res. 1983, 43, 5006-5009.
6. Leyland-Jones, B.; Donnelly, H.; Groshen, S.; Myskowski, P.;
    Donner, A. L.; Fanucchi, M.; Fox, J. J. J. Infectious Dis.
    1986, 154, 430-436.
7. Fanucchi, M. P.; Leyland-Jones, B.; Young, C. W.; Burchenal, J.
    H.; Watanabe, K. A.; Fox, J. J. Cancer Treatment Rep. 1985, 69,
    55-59.
8. Watanabe, K. A.; Su, T-L.; Reichman, U.; Greenberg, N.; Lopez,
    C.; Fox, J. J. J. Med. Chem. 1984, 27, 91-94.
9. Perlman, M. E.; Watanabe, K. A.; Schinazi, R. F.; Fox, J. J.
    J. Med. Chem. 1985, 28, 741-748.

10. Fox, J. J.; Watanabe, K. A.; Schinazi, R. F.; Lopez, C.   In
    Herpes Viruses and Virus Chemotherapy; Kano, R.; Nakajima, A.,
    Eds.; Excerpta Medica: Amsterdam, 1985; pp 53-56.   Based upon
    proceedings of International Symposium on Pharmacological and
    Clinical Approaches to Herpes Viruses and Virus chemotherapy
    presented in Oiso, Japan, September, 1984.
11. Schinazi, R. F.; Peters, J.; Sokol, M. K.; Nahmias, A. J.
    Antimicrobial Agents Chemother. 1983, 24, 95-103.
12. Chou, T-C.; Kong, X-B.; Potter, V. P.; Schmid, F. A.; Fox, J. J.;
    Watanabe, K. A.; Fanucchi, M.   Proc. Amer. Assoc. Cancer Res.,
    1985, 26, 333.
13. Chou, T-C.; Kong, X-B.; Fanucchi, M. P.; Cheng, Y-C.; Takahashi,
    K.; Watanabe, K. A.; Fox, J. J.   Antimicrobial Agents Chemother.
    1987, 31, 1355-1358.
14. Cheng, Y-C.; Dutschman, G.; Fox, J. J.; Watanabe, K. A.; Machida,
    H.   Antimicrobial Agents Chemother. 1981, 20, 420-423.
15. Lopez, C.; Watanabe, K. A.; Fox, J. J.   Antimicrobial Agents
    Chemother. 1980, 17, 803-806.
16. Mansuri, M. M.; Ghazzouli, I.; Chen, M. S.; Howel, H. G.;
    Brodfuehrer, P. R.; Benigni, D. A.; Martin, J. C.   J. Med. Chem.
    1987, 30, 867-871.
17. Machida, H.; Kuninaka, A.; Yoshino, H.   Antimicrobial Agents
    Chemother. 1982, 21, 358-361.
18. Soike, K. F.; Cantrell, C.; Gerone, P. J.   Ibid., 1986, 29, 20-
    25.
19. Blumberg, B. S.; London, W. T.   In Clinical Management of
    Gastrointestinal Cancer; Decosse, J. J.; Sherlock, P., Eds.; Martinus
    Nijhoff Publishers: Boston, 1984; pp. 71-91.
20. Galibert, F.; Chen, T. V.; Mandart, E.   Proc. Natl. Acad. Sci.
    U.S.A., 1981, 78, 5315-5319.
21. Blumberg, B. S.   Hum. Pathol. 1981, 12, 1107-1113.
22. Kaplan, P. M.; Greenman, R. I.; Gerin, J. L.; Purcell, R. H.;
    Robinson, W. S.   J. Virol. 1973, 12, 995-1005.
23. Hantz, O.; Ooka, T.; Vitvitski, L.; Pichoud, C.; Trepo, C.
    Antimicrobial Agents Chemother. 1984, 25, 242-246.
24. Hantz, O.; Allaudeen, H. S.; Ooka, T.; De Clercq, E.; Trepo, C.
    Antiviral Res. 1984, 4, 187-199.
25. Fourel, I.; Hantz, O.; Watanabe, K. A.; Fox, J. J.; Trepo, C.
    Hepatology 1987, 7, 1122.

RECEIVED January 15, 1988

Chapter 11

Fluorinated Analogs of Cell-Surface Carbohydrates as Potential Chemotherapeutic Agents

Moheswar Sharma, Ralph J. Bernacki, and Walter Korytnyk

Department of Experimental Therapeutics, Grace Cancer Drug Center, Roswell Park Memorial Institute, 666 Elm Street, Buffalo, NY 14263

The rationale for designing fluorinated analogs of cell surface carbohydrates as anticancer agents is described. Using diethylaminosulfur trifluoride, a general and a convenient method for synthesis of 6-deoxy-6-fluoro-hexosamines and 9-deoxy-9-fluoro-N-acetylneuraminic acid has been developed. This reagent has also been used to introduce geminal fluorine both in the 6-position and 4-position (6,6-difluoro-D-galactose and 4,4-difluoro-N-acetyl-D-glucosamine). Another method for incorporation of fluorine is the addition of fluorine to the double bond in the acetylated glycals using XeF_2 in the presence of BF_3. This process is shown to be a convenient route to synthesize 1,2-dideoxy-1,2-difluoro sugars and 2-deoxy-2,3-di-fluoro-N-acetyl-D-neuraminic acid. Conventional methods of fluorination are used to synthesize 6-deoxy-6-fluoro-D-galactosamine and 4-deoxy-4-fluoro-D-galactosamine. The effects of these analogs on the growth of tumor cells (in vitro) and inhibition of macromolecular biosynthesis, as well as their therapeutic activity on syngenic mice with ascites L1210 leukemia (in vivo) are reported.

As part of our program on antitumor plasma-membrane modifiers and inhibitors, we have synthesized several carbohydrate analogs, substituting a fluorine for a hydroxyl group. These analogs were designed to act as carbohydrate chain terminators of cell surface glycoconjugates or as inhibitors of various enzymes involved in glycoprotein metabolism. Alteration of the cell surface carbohydrates could be achieved either by inhibition of

NOTE: This chapter is dedicated to the late Walter Korytnyk.

0097–6156/88/0374–0191$06.00/0
© 1988 American Chemical Society

their biosynthesis or by incorporation of modified derivatives. This could result in significant changes in the membrane structure. The chemical synthesis of the fluorinated derivatives of cell sur- face carbohydrates, namely galactose, L-fucose, galactosamine, glucosamine, mannosamine and N-acetyl-D-neuraminic acid as well as their biological effects will be reviewed in the context of ongoing research in this area.

There has been considerable interest to pursue approaches directed towards the modification and inhibition of cell-surface glycoprotein. Such modification may change the immunogenicity, tumorogenicity and/or metastatic potential of cancer cells. The primary target of such modification are membrane sialic acid, amino sugars, and the other cell-surface neutral sugars. In addition, some carbohydrate analogs are expected to modify the nucleotide pool sizes and hence have potential use in combination chemotherapy with nucleoside analogs. Plasma-membrane components are involved in cell growth, division, movement, communication, differentiation and antigenicity. Extensive investigation has shown that changes occur in these cell-surface properties following oncogenic trans- formation by viruses or carcinogens (1-3). One of the major com- ponents of the cell surface found to be altered following transfor- mation are the glycoconjugates. The glycoconjugates comprise glycoproteins and glycolipids that are attached by their hydro- phobic region to the lipid bilayer. The carbohydrate chains of these molecules are found on the outer surface of the plasma mem- brane and consist of (a) amino sugars, N-acetyl-D-glucosamine (GlcNAc), N-acetyl-D-galactosamine (GalNAc) and N-acetyl-D-neura- minic acid (NANA); (b) neutral sugars like L-fucose, D-mannose and D-galactose. The attachment to membrane protein occurs either as GlcNAc-asparagine linked N-glycosidically or as GalNAc-serine (or threonine) which are linked O-glycosidically. L-Fucose and sialic acids generally occur as the terminal sugar (4). This complexity confers a good deal of informational potential to the surface car- bohydrate present in the various branched oligosaccharide struc- tures (5).

The rationale to pursue studies on the synthesis and biochemis- try of fluorosugars is based on the observations that: I. Bio- chemical differences exist in the cell surface complex carbohy- drates of tumor cells. II. Sialic acids may mask cell-surface antigen; its removal enhances cellular immunogenicity. III. Carbo- hydrates are involved in the social behavior of cells such as cell to cell communications resulting in contact inhibition. IV. Changes in cell surface carbohydrates are found to effect the uptake of drugs and nutrients. V. Differences are found to develop in the metabolism of membrane sugar following oncogenic transformation. VI. Some membrane sugar and their analogs are cytotoxic to tumor cells (6). VII. Uptake and accumulation of some membrane sugars results in the lowering of specific intracellular nucleotide pools. VIII. Some membrane sugars and their analogs have been shown to inhibit envelope DNA and RNA virus proliferation. IX. Membrane signal transduction is altered by oncogene products fol- lowing transformation.

The membrane sugar analogs under development in this program, may act on tumor or virally infected cells in the following manner:

(a) In competition as an antimetabolite with the natural sugar substrate leading to the inhibition of membrane glycoconjugate formation. (b) Via incorporation of structurally similar analogs into glyconjugate leading to chain termination. (c) In conjugation with specific nucleotides leading to an alteration in nucleotide pool sizes (potential use in combination chemotherapy). (d) Through introduction of changes in cell surface antigenicity and immunogenicity. (e) By modification of the social behavior of cells leading to decreased tumor growth and metastasis. (f) Antiviral activity.

Synthesis of Fluorinated Membrane Sugar Analogs

Fully acetylated membrane sugars and their analogs are found to be more cytotoxic than their corresponding unacetylated derivatives. These differences may have been the result of an increase in the agents cellular permeability and passive uptake, since it has been found that fully acetylated glucosamine (β-PAGlcNAc) has a higher octanol/water partition coefficient (0.42) than the parent compound, N-acetyl-D-glucosamine (0.17). After intracellular uptake, PA-GTcNAc was O-deacetylated, phosphorylated, and activated to form UDP-GlcNAc, resulting in a significant lowering of cellular UTP and CTP pools (6).

A general and convenient method for the synthesis of 6-deoxy-6-fluorohexoses has been developed using the fluorinating agent N,N-diethylaminosulfur trifluoride (DAST) (7). This reagent permits the use of the acetyl as the protecting group; however, the reaction also runs smoothly when the protecting groups are benzyl or methyl ethers as well (8). DAST also dispenses with the necessity of introducing a leaving group as the hydroxyl group is being directly replaced with fluorine. The following 6-deoxy-6-fluoro hexopyranoses have been prepared using this reagent from the 6-hydroxy-acetylated hexoses: D-glucose, N-acetyl-D-glucosamine, N-acetyl-D-galactosamine and N-acetyl-D-mannosamine. In the preparation of 6-deoxy-6-fluoro-D-mannosamine from 6-deoxy-6-fluoro-D-glucosamine by base epimerization of the N-acetyl-derivative, the separation was very difficult for large-scale preparations, even though the epimeric mixture contained about 20% of the D-mannoepimer. We resorted, therefore, to the use of N-acetyl-D-mannosamine (9). The usual procedure for the preparation of the 6-hydroxy-tetraacetyl-derivative could not be applied with N-acetyl-D-mannosamine as the initial tritylation step involved partial epimerization to N-acetyl-D-glucosamine in the presence of pyridine. The starting material was 2-acetamido-1,3-di-O-acetyl-2-deoxy-4,6-O-isopropylidene-D-manno-pyranose (1) (10). The acetal group was opened up with aqueous acetic acid (60%) to give (2) (Figure 1) and the primary hydroxyl group was tritylated in the usual way to give (3). The hydroxyl group in the 4-position was acetylated and the trityl group was removed to yield (4) which was then fluorinated with DAST in anhydrous diglyme to give (5).

Anhydrous diglyme was also used as the solvent in the preparation of 6-deoxy-6-fluoro-D-galactose (11) and 6-deoxy-6,6-difluoro-D-galactose (8) (Lee, H.H.; Hodgson, P.G.; Bernacki, R.J.; Korytnyk, W.; Sharma, M. Carbohydr. Res., in press) (34) from 1,2:3,4-di-O-isopropylidene-α-D-galactose and 1,2:3,4-di-O-isopropylidene-α-D-galactohexo-dialdo-1,5-pyranose (6) respectively, by treatment with DAST. Deblocking of the intermediate difluoro deri-

vative (7) to give the target compound (8) was accomplished by conventional acid hydrolysis (Figure 2). Similarly, the preparation of
the 6-deoxy-6-fluoro-L-galactose or 6-fluoro-L-fucose, from 1,2:
3,4-di-O-isopropylidene-L-galactopyranose (12) has been reported
(13).
    Fluorination of N-acetyl-D-galactosamine by treatment of 1,3,4-
tri-O-acetyl-N-acetyl-D-galactosamine with DAST gave low yields of
the desired product. An alternative procedure was adopted to prepare 6-deoxy-6-fluoro-N-acetyl-D-galactosamine (11) (14). Treatment of benzyl 2-acetamido-2-deoxy-3,4-O-isopropylidene-6-O-mesyl-α-
D-galactopyranoside (9) (Figure 3) with cesium fluoride in boiling
ethanediol gave (10) which was deblocked by catalytic hydrogenolysis to (11) and then acetylated to (12).
    Fluorination of the anomeric carbon atom along with the adjacent
carbon atom, occurs by the action of fluorine on acetylated glycals
(15). Another method of fluorination of acetylated glycals is the
use of trifluoromethyl hypofluorite (CF₃OF) (16,17), which results in a side product of trifluoromethyl glycoside. We are using
xenon difluoride (18), a reagent that can be handled without spe-
cial care or apparatus. The convenience of this reagent allows the
preparation of ^{18}F-labelled compounds and hence is of potential
use in positron emmission tomography. Boron trifluoride-etherate
was carefully used as a mild acid catalyst to effect the fluorination and benzene-ether mixture as a solvent to avoid dimeric and
polymeric products. Thus, 3,4,6-tri-O-acetyl-2-deoxy-2-fluoro-α-D-
glucopyranosyl fluoride (14), 3,4,6-tri-O-acetyl-2-deoxy-2-fluoro-β-
D-glucopyranosyl fluoride (15) and 3,4,6-tri-O-acetyl-2-deoxy-2-
fluoro-β-D-mannopyranosyl fluoride (16) were all obtained by fluorination of 3,4,6-tri-O-acetyl-D-glucal (13) with xenon difluoride
(Figure 4) through both cis and trans addition of fluorine (19).
The same mode of reaction was observed with tri-O-acetyl galactal.
    The composition of products resulting from cis and trans
addition of fluorine was found to be the same when the reaction was
carried out in an oxygen or nitrogen atmosphere to avoid any free-
radical reaction mechanism. This reaction with 3,4-di-O-acetyl-
L-fucal (17) (20) gave almost exclusively the single addition product 3,4-di-O-acetyl-1,2-dideoxy-1,2-difluoro-L-fucose (18)(19),
which on acid hydrolysis gave 2-deoxy-L-fucose (19) (Figure 5).
From our experimental data it appears that the reaction proceeds as
shown in Figure 6.
    The reaction of unsaturated sialic acid with xenon difluoride
was also studied in the similar fashion (Figure 7). Methyl 4,7,8,9-
tetra-O-acetyl-2,3-dehydro-2-deoxy-N-acetylneuraminate (20)(21) reacted with xenon difluoride in methylene chloride in the presence
of boron trifluorideetherate in an oxygen atmosphere to give the
2,3-difluoro-derivative (21). In the absence of oxygen the reaction was very sluggish and considerable decomposition occurred.
The acetylated 2,3-difluoro-methylester (21) was deacetylated to
the corresponding difluoro acid (22) at pH 7 without loss of fluorine. The latter compound on acid hydrolysis gave the 3-fluoro-N-
acetylneuraminic acid (23) with the hydrolytic removal of anomeric
fluorine. This process significantly improved the yield of 3-
fluoro-N-acetylneuraminic acid over the previously reported proce-

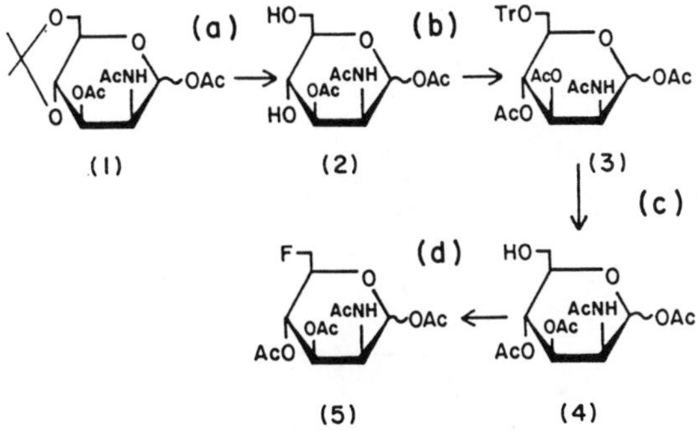

Figure 1. Synthesis of tetra-0-acetyl-6-deoxy-6-fluoro-D-mannosamine (5). (a) AeOH-H_2O, 50%, (b) tritylation, Ac_2O/Py. (c) Pd/c-AcOH, [H]$_2$ (d) DAST.

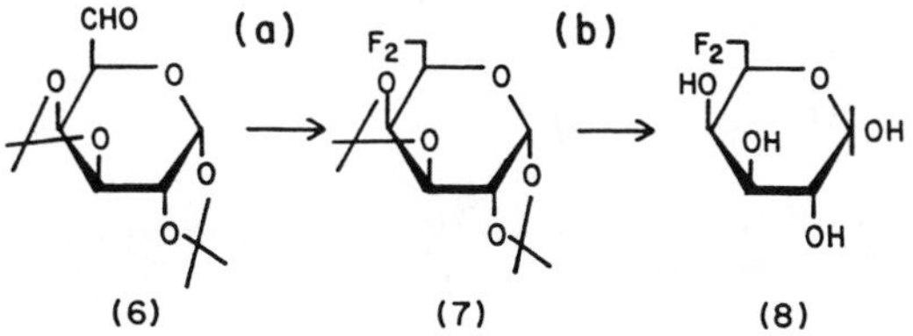

Figure 2. Synthesis of 6-deoxy-6,6-difluoro-D-galactose (8). (a) DAST-CH_2Cl_2, (b) AcOH-H_2O, 80%, 90°C.

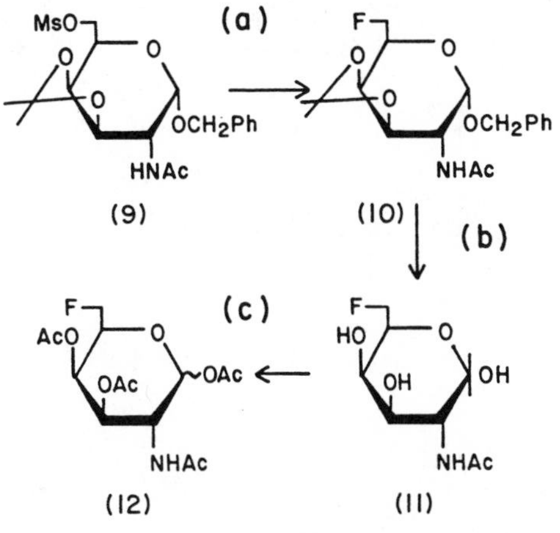

Figure 3. Scheme for synthesis of N-acetyl-3,4-di-0-acetyl-6-deoxy-6-fluoro-Dgalactosamine (11). (a) CsF/ethylene-glycol (200°C), (b) Pd/C in AcOH, [H], (c) Ac_2O/Py.

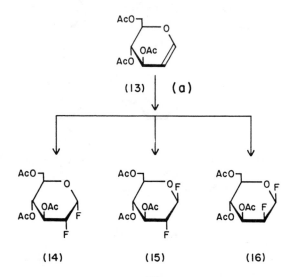

Figure 4. Fluorination of tri-O-acetyl-D-glucal with XeF$_2$.
(a) XeF$_2$, BF$_3$ etherate, (14)61%, (15)12%, (16)5%.

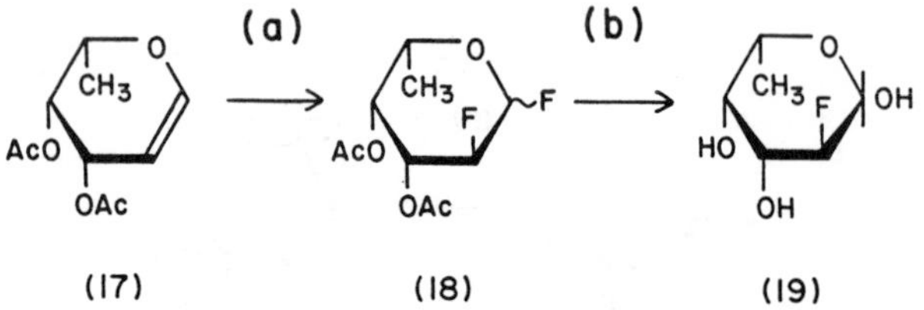

Figure 5. Synthesis of 2-deoxy-2-fluoro-L-fucose (19).
(a) XeF$_2$, BF$_3$-etherate, (b) 0.5 M HCl.

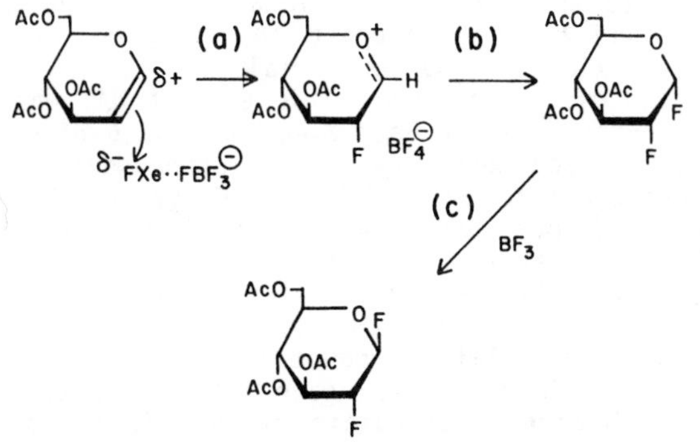

Figure 6. Possible mechanism of addition of fluorine to glycals with XeF_2. (a) Electrophilic addition of F from XeF_2-BF_3 complex, (b) addition of F on carboxonium ion, (c) anomerization of pyranoxylfluoride with BF_3.

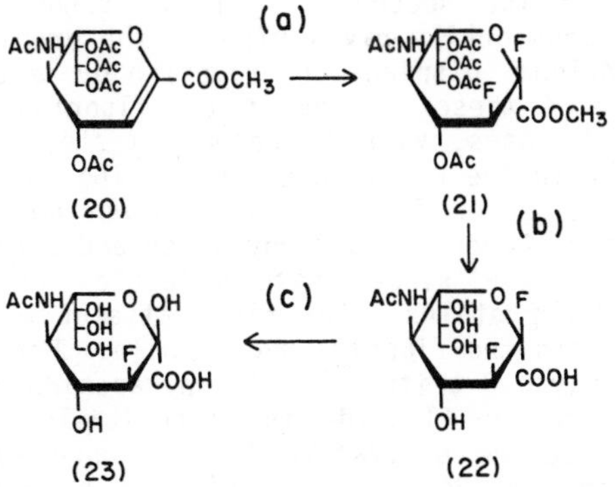

Figure 7. Synthesis of 3-deoxy-3-fluoro-NANA (23). (a) XeF_2, BF_3-etherate, (b) NaOMe-MEOH, (c) 0.5 N HCl.

dure (22). The ^{19}F-NMR data were used to determine the con-figuration of the fluorine atom of methyl 4,7,8,9-tetra-0-acetyl-2-deoxy-2,3-difluoro-N-acetylneuraminic acid (21). The magnitude of the $J_{F-2,F-3}$ (19.5 Hz) indicates an axial-equitorial arrange-ment. The coupling constant $J_{F-2,H-3}$ (19.5 Hz) indicates a di-axial orientation of the anomeric fluorine and the H-3. These coupling constants and the absence of any long range coupling be-tween fluorine and hydrogen suggest the ring conformation to be $^{2}C_5$ (D) with F-2 axial and F-3 equitorial.

The 9-position of N-acetylneuraminic acid (NANA) was substituted following two routes: Figure 8a, 2-Acetamido-2,6-dideoxy-6-fluoro-D-glucopyranose (24) (8,23) was condensed with potassium di-tert-butyloxaloacetate (Sharma, M.; Korytnyk, W., Carbohydr. Res., in press) and subsequently hydrolyzed to 9-deoxy-9-fluoro-NANA. Figure 8b, Methyl 2-0-methyl-4,7,8-tri-0-benzyl-N-acetyl-neuraminate (30) was obtained by benzylation of methyl 2-0-methyl-9-0-trityl-N-acetylneuraminate (28) and followed by detritylation. Treatment of the detritylated product (30) with DAST, followed by hydrogenolysis and hydrolysis, gave the 9-deoxy-9-fluoro-NANA (27). The detritylated intermediate product (30) was oxidized at the 9-position to the corresponding 9-aldehyde derivative (31) and then converted to the 9-deoxy-9-difluoro-N-acetylneuraminic acid derivative (32). The ^{13}C NMR spectrum of 9-deoxy-9-fluoro-NANA (27) showed that the introduction of fluorine at the 9-position deshielded C-9 from δ63.5 p.p.m. to 81.4 (as a doublet J_{C-F} 164.9 Hz). The ^{19}F NMR spectrum of 9-deoxy-9-fluoro-NANA gave a clear sextet (-235.4 p.p.m., $J_{F, H-9}$, 46.8 Hz; $J_{F, H-8}$, 26.0 Hz) in-dicating the absence of any anomeric isomer.

Substitution of the secondary hydroxyl group of carbohydrates with fluorine occassionally gives rise to the problem of inversion, both in a conventional displacement reaction or reaction with DAST. However, the use of these methods in the fluorination reaction are workable, in such cases, with a preceeding step of inversion when necessary, to obtain the required epimeric fluorinated product (24, 25). We were interested in introducing fluorine in the C-4 posi-tion of 2-acetamido-2-deoxy-D-glucopyranose and 2-acetamido-2-deoxy-D-galactopyranose since these molecules occur in the core region of the glycoproteins. Our first attempt was the opening of the 3,4-epoxide with the fluoride nucleophile. Benzyl 2-acetamido-3,4-anhydro-2-deoxy-6-0-trityl-α-D-glucopyranoside (33) was treated with tetrabutylammonium fluoride in acetonitrile to give the cor-responding D-gulosamine derivative (26) (Figure 9). Inversion of the hydroxyl group of (34) at C-3 could not be achieved to obtain the D-galactosamine derivative. However, 2-acetamido-1,3,6-tri-0-acetyl-2,4-dideoxy-4-fluoro-D-gulose (35) was isolated and showed encouraging inhibitory activity on the growth of L1210 leukemia cells.

2-Acetamido-2,4-dideoxy-4-fluoro-D-galactopyranose (38) and 2-acetamido-2,4,6-trideoxy-4,6-difluoro-D-galactopyranose (43) were synthesized from benzyl 2-acetamido-3,4-di-0-benzyl-2-deoxy-4-0-mesyl-α-D-glucopyranoside (36) and benzyl 2-acetamido-3-0-benzyl-2-deoxy-4,6-di-0-mesyl-α-D-glucopyranoside (41) (Figure 10), re-spectively, by displacement of the methanesulphonyloxy groups with tetrabutylammonium fluoride. These fluoro sugar derivatives were

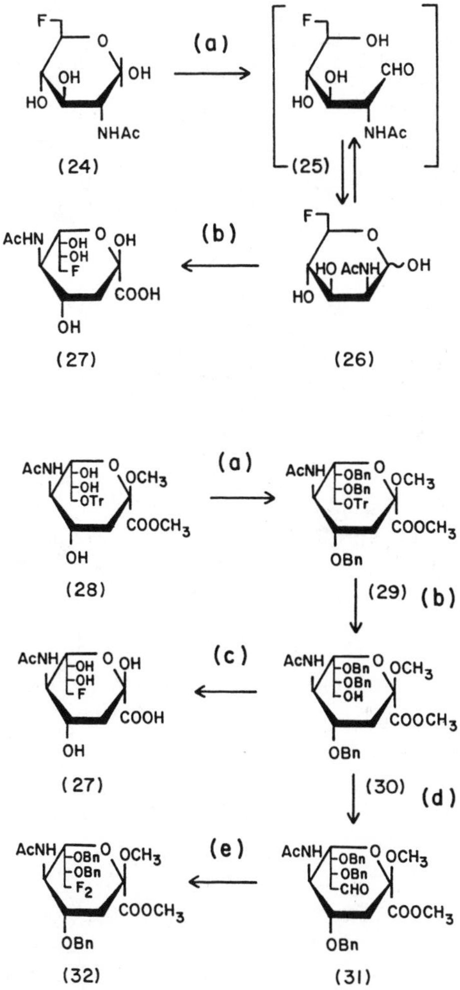

Figure 8. Top, synthesis of 9-deoxy-9-fluoro-NANA from 6-deoxy-6-fluoro-N-acetyl-D-glucosamine (27). (a) Potassium di-tert-butyl-oxaloacetate-MEOH (epimerization), (b) condensation and hydrolysis. Bottom, synthesis of 9-deoxy-9-fluoro-NANA from NANA (27). (a) Benzyl bromide-Ba(OH)$_2$-DMF, (b) AcOH-H$_2$O (70%), 90 °C, (c) DAST-CH$_2$Cl$_2$, NaOH-H$_2$O, 0.05 N HCl, (d) Py-CrO$_3$-CH$_2$Cl$_2$, (e) DAST-CH$_2$Cl$_2$.

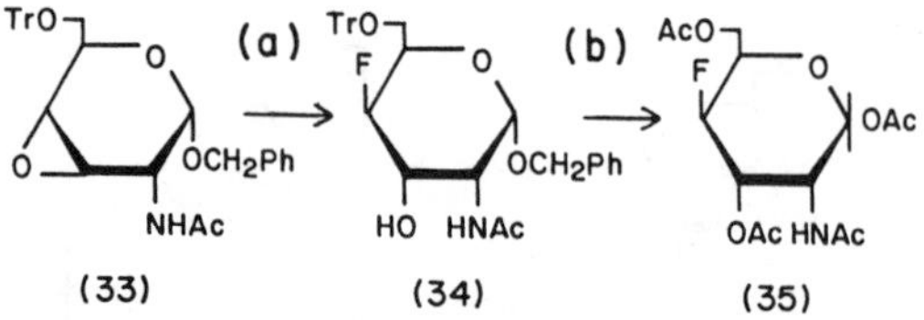

Figure 9. Synthesis of N-acetyl-1,3,6-tri-O-acetyl 4-deoxy-4-fluoro-D-gulosamine (35). (a) Bu$_4$NF-CH$_3$CN, (b) Pd/C-AcOH [H], Py/AcOH.

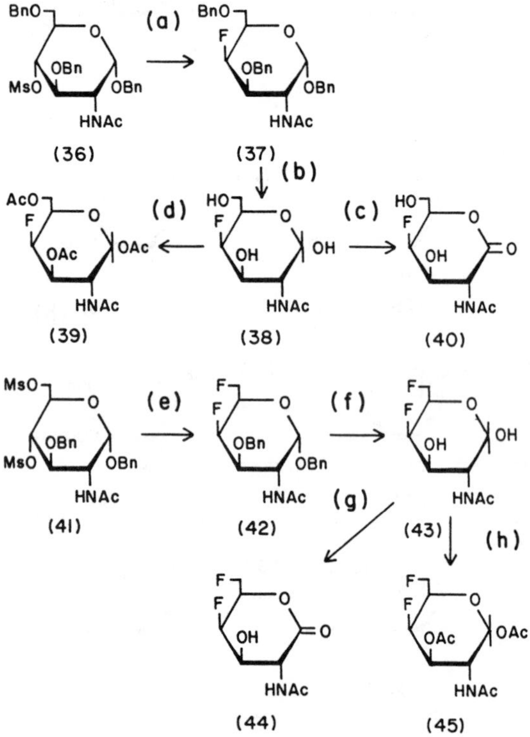

Figure 10. Scheme for synthesis of N-acetyl-4-deoxy-4-fluoro and N-acetyl-4,6-dideoxy-4,6-difluoro-D-galactosamine (39) and (45). (a) Bu$_4$NF-CH$_3$CN, (b) [H], Pd/c-AcOH, (c) Pt/C-H$_2$O-O$_2$, (d) Ac$_2$O/Py, (e) Bu$_4$NF-CH$_3$CN, (f) [H], Pd/C-AcOH, (g)Pt/C-H$_2$O-O$_2$, (h) Ac$_2$O-Py.

also obtained by treating benzyl 2-acetamido-3,6-di-O-benzyl-2-deoxy-α-D-glucopyranoside and benzyl 2-acetamido-3-O-benzyl-α-D-glucopyranoside (27-29) with DAST in methylene chloride, but in much lower yield. The intermediates were deprotected by hydrogenolysis to give the fluorinated sugars (38) and (43). The aldonolactones (40) and (44) derived from these sugars by oxidation with molecular oxygen in the presence of platinum on activated charcoal were found to be strong inhibitors (Ki 27.2 μM and 41.4 μM, respectively) of hexosaminidases (25,32). The acetylated derivatives of these sugars (39) and (45) were shown to be very good antitumor agents in tissue culture (Table I). In the ^{19}F NMR spectrum of the 4,6-dideoxy-4,6-difluoro-galactosamine derivative (42), it appeared from the vicinal coupling constants ($J_{F-6, H-5}$ 12.30 Hz) that the favored rotamer about the C-5-C-6 has F-6 anti- periplanar to C-4-C-5.

The biological activity of these fluoro sugars suggested the preparation of the 4-deoxy-4,4-difluoro (48) and 3-deoxy-3-fluoro-N-acetyl-D-glucosamine derivatives. Benzyl-2-acetamido-3,6-di-O-benzyl-2-deoxy-α-D-xylo-4-uloside (46) (Figure 11) was treated with DAST to give the 4-deoxy-4,4-difluoro-D-glucosamine derivative (47) in very good yield. After deprotection and acetylation the difluoro compound (48) showed very good inhibitory activity of cell growth (L1210) in vitro (Table I). 2-Acetamido-1,3,6-tri-O-acetyl-2,4-dideoxy-4-fluoro-D-glucosamine (52) was synthesized by double inversion at the 4-position following the scheme as shown in Figure 12. Compound (49) was obtained from (36) by treatment with lithium benzoate in hot N,N-dimethylformamide, followed by debenzoylation with Amberlyst A-26-(OH) resin in methanol. Treatment of (49) with DAST and subsequent hydrogenolysis gave 2-acetamido-2,4-dideoxy-4-fluoro-D-glucosamine (51) which was acetylated to (52).

Biological Activity of Fluorinated Carbohydrates

In view of the physico-chemical properties of the CF bond, which by size falls between the CH and C-OH bond, its introduction into carbohydrates should result in biologically analogous molecules. Numerous biochemical applications of fluorosugars have appeared in the earlier literature (30,31), and these studies prompted the development of several fluorosugars within this program. A number of these sugars have been tested for their effect on tumor cell growth in vitro, their effects on macromolecular biosynthesis and their antitumor activity in mice. These preliminary studies demonstrate that the fluorosugars as a group are biologically active. Their addition at concentrations ranging from $10^{-3}M$ to $10^{-6}M$ (Table I) to L1210 leukemia cultures resulted in cell growth inhibition. Generally, the fully acetylated compounds having greater lipophilicity were more cytotoxic to cells. The nonacetylated agents, 6-F-D-galactose and 9-F-NANA demonstrated cell growth inhibition at higher concentration, 1.0 and 0.8 mM, respectively. These two agents in addition demonstrated an ability to alter cellular sialic acid metabolism. Thus, 6-F-D-galactose treatment resulted in decreased L1210 leukemia cell ectosialyltransferase activity (34) while 9-F-NANA was found to act as a substrate for CMP-NANA synthetase (Petrie, C.R.; Sharma, M.; simmons, O.D.; Korytnyk, W., unpublished results 1987) and thus serves as a precursor for membrane incorporation.

The fluorinated neutral sugars also mimicked their parent sugars by competing with them for incorporation into macromolecular components (Table II). 6-F-D-Galactose and 6-F-L-fucose specifically decreased the incorporation of their corresponding parent sugar to 39 and 9%, respectively, in murine P288 lymphoma cells grown in tissue culture. Little specific effect was noted on leukemia cell incorporation of glcNAc or leucine (leu) with these two agents, while fully acetylated sugars reduced the incorporation of all precursors, nonselectively (Table II). The administration of fluorosugars to mice with L1210 leukemia resulted, in all cases, with small increases in life span (% ILS), ranging from 11 to 68% (Table III). The most active agent, 4-F-galNAc-tri-O-acetate or flugal (68% ILS) is currently being evaluated in mice with various other tumors to more fully assess its antitumor potential.

Table I. Effects of Fluoro-Sugar Analogs on Murine L1210 Leukemia
Cell Growth in vitro

Fluoro Sugar	IC_{50}, M* Leukemia L1210
6-F-GlcNAc-tri-O-acetate	5.0×10^{-5}
6-F-ManNAc-tri-O-acetate	1.0×10^{-4}
6-F-GalNAc-tri-O-acetate	1.7×10^{-4}
6-F-GulNAc-tri-O-acetate	6.0×10^{-5}
6-F-4-ene-lyxNAc-di-O-acetate	1.0×10^{-4}
6-F-4-ene-lyx-tri-O-acetate	3.2×10^{-6}
6-F-Gal (34)	1.0×10^{-3}
6-F-Mann-tetra-O-acetate	5.5×10^{-5}
6-F-Glc-tetra-O-acetate	5.0×10^{-5}
4-F-GalNAc-tri-O-acetate (flugal)	3.0×10^{-5}
4,4-Di-F-GlcNAc-tri-O-acetate	3.4×10^{-5}
4,6-Di-F-GalNAc-di-O-acetate	2.0×10^{-5}
4-F-GlcNAc-Tri-O-acetate	3.0×10^{-5}
9-F-NANA	3.6×10^{-4}
9-F-NANA	8.0×10^{-4} (TA3)

*The concentration of fluorosugar which inhibited murine L1210 leukemia cell growth in culture by 50% over a two-day period (33). Cultures were inoculated with 5×10^4 cells/mL in RPMI 1640 medium containing 10% fetal bovine serum. Sugar analogs were added and growth allowed for 24 h. Cell number was measured and % control (no sugar analog added) growth was calculated. The IC_{50} (50% growth inhibitory concentration) was determined from the dose response curve. All assays were performed in duplicate on at least two separate occassions. TA3:Mouse mammary adenocarcinoma.

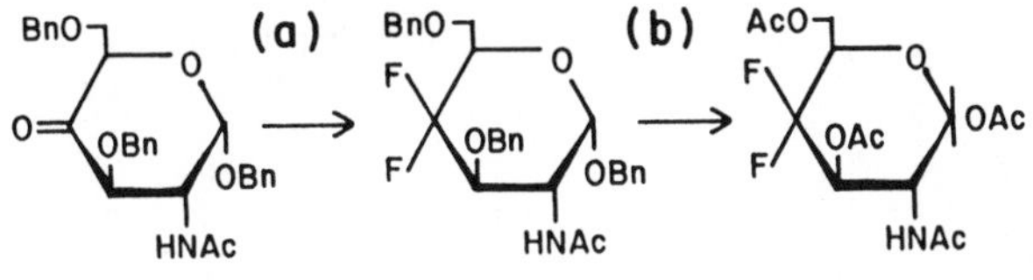

Figure 11.   Synthesis of N-acetyl-1,3,6-tri-O-acetyl-4-deoxy-4,4-difluoro glucosamine (48).   (a) DAST-CH$_2$Cl$_2$, (b) [H], Pd/C-ACOH, Ac$_2$O-Py.

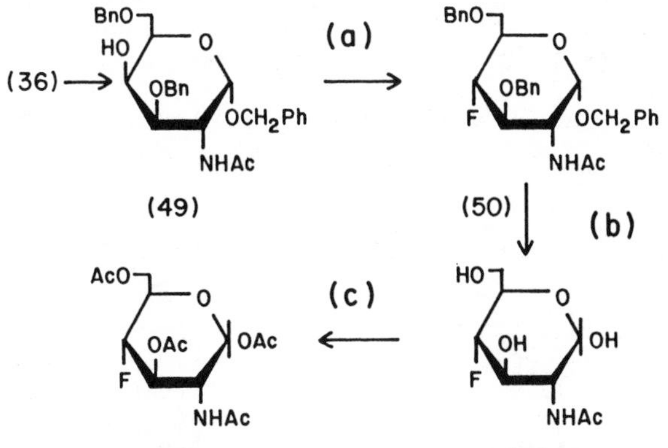

Figure 12.   Synthesis of N-acetyl-1,3,6-tri-O-acetyl-4-deoxy-4-fluoro-D-glucosamine (52).   (a) DAST-CH$_2$Cl$_2$, (b) [H], Pd/C-AcOH, (c) Ac$_2$O-Py.

Table II. Effects of Fluoro-Sugars on Macromolecular Biosynthesis in
P288 Lymphoma Cells

Fluoro-Sugars,	Conc. [M]	P288 Lymphoma Incorporation, of [3H] Sugars and Leu % Control**			
		L-Fuc*	Gal*	GlcNac*	Leu*
6-F-Gal (14)	10⁻³	-	39	89	84
6-F-L-Fucose (14)	10⁻³	9	-	88	
6-F-Glc-β-tri-O-acetate,	10⁻³		-	46	51
6-F-ManNAc-tri-O-acetate,	10⁻³		-	55	71
4-F-GalNAc-tri-O-acetate,	10⁻⁵		-	88	86
6-F-Mann	10⁻³		-	-	-

**P288 lymphoma cells (10⁵ cells/mL) were inoculated in medium RPMI 1640 containing 10% FBS (fetal bovine serum) with the indicated [3H] radiolabeled precursor* (1 μCi/mL). After 5 h the amount of incorporated radioactivity was determined and compared with control. All assays were performed in duplicate on three separate occassions and the results listed are means.

Table III. Effects of Fluoro-Sugars on L1210 Leukemia in Mice in
vivo *

Fluoro-Sugar	Tumor	Dose(mg/kg)	%ILS
6-F-GlcNAc-tri-O-acetate	L1210	6.25	12.2
6-F-Mann-tri-O-acetate	L1210	25.0	11.5
4,6-Di-F-GalNAc-tri-O-acetate	L1210	10.0	11.4
4-F-GlcNAc-tri-O-acetate	L1210	100.0	33.0
6-F-Mann	L1210	200.0	17.8
6-F-Mann-tetra-O-acetate	L1210	200.0	27.4
6-F Gal	L1210	25.0	32.0
4-F-GalNAc-tri-O-acetate (Flugal) (30)	L1210	50.0	68.0
4-F-GulNAc-tri-O-acetate	L1210	50.0	12.2
9-F-NANA	L1210	50.0	19.0
6-F-Glc-tetra-O-acetate	L1210	6.25	21.0
1,2-Di-F-Glc-tri-O-acetate	L1210	400.0	35.0

*DBA/2 (Dilute Brown non-Agouti) female mice (19-20 g) were inoculated i.p. with 10⁶ L1210 leukemia cells on day zero. Starting on day one mice were given various dosages (5 mice/dosage level) of the test agent i.p., once per day through day 5. Life span was checked daily. The % measure in lifespan (% ILS) was calculated as compared to the control group, consisting of 8-10 animals. The optimum % ILS is listed.

Conclusions and Future Studies
This program has attempted to demonstrate that, by interfering or modifying the biosynthesis of components of tumor cell surface glycoconjugates, development of chemotherapeutic agents may result. In pursuing this avenue several analogs of cell-surface carbohydrates were synthesized and tested both in vitro and in vivo as antitumor agents. Combination chemotherapy with nucleoside analogs also may improve the therapeutic response as noted with D-glucosamine and penta-0-acetyl-β-D-glucosamine (β-PAGlcNAc) in combination with azaribine (33). It appears from the preliminary experimental data in our laboratory and others that fluorinated sugar analogs are membrane-active agents and are worth further synthetic and biochemical investigation.

Acknowledgments
We would like to thank Dr. E. Mihich for his active encouragement throughout the program. We would also like to thank Dr. B. Paul and Mr. N.J. Angelino for their active support in the program. This study was supported by CA24538, CA13038 and CA42898 from the National Cancer Institute.

LITERATURE CITED

1. Nicolson, G.L. Biochem. Biophys. Acta. 1976, 458, 1-72.
2. Nicolson, G.L.; Poste, G; New England J. Med. 1976, 295 197-203;253-258.
3. Poste, G, Weiss, L. "Fundamental Aspects of Metastasis", Weiss, L., Ed.; North Holland Publishing Co., Amsterdam 1976, p. 25.
4. Hughes, R.C. "Membrane Glycoproteins". Butterworth, London-Boston, 1976.
5. Winzler, R.J. In "Membrane Mediated Information". Kent, P.W., Ed., Medical and Technical Publishing Co. Ltd., 1973, Vol. 1, p. 3-19.
6. Bernacki, R.J.; Sharma, M.; Porter, N.K.; Rustum, Y.; Paul, B.; Korytnyk, W. J. Supramol. Structure, 1978, 7, 235-250.
7. Middleton, W.J., J. Org. Chem., 1975, 40, 574-578.
8. Sharma, M.; Korytnyk, W. Tetrahedron Lett. 1977, 573-576.
9. Sharma, M.; Korytnyk, W. Carbohydr. Res. 1980, 83, 163-169.
10. Hasegawa, A.; Fletcher, H.G. Carbohydr. Res. 1973, 29, 209-222.
11. Taylor, N.F.; Kent, P.W. J. Chem. Soc. 1958, 872-875.
12. Fush, H.L.; Isbell, H.S. Methods Carbohydr. Chem. 1962, 1, 127-130.
13. Sufrin, J.R.; Bernacki, R.J.; Morin, M.J.; Korytnyk, W. J. Med. Chem. 1980, 23, 143-149.
14. Sharma, M.; Potti, P.G.; Simmons, O.; Korytnyk, W. Carbohydr. Res. 1987, 162, 41-52.
15. Ido, T.; Wan, C.N.; Fowler, J.S.; Wolf, A.P. J. Org. Chem. 1977, 42, 2341-2342.
16. Adamson, J.; Mercus, D.M. Carbohydr. Res. 1970, 13, 314-316.
17. Butchard, G.C.; Kent, P.W. Tetrahedron 1979, 35, 2551-2554.
18. Greigorcic, A.; Zupan, M. J. Org. Chem. 1979, 44, 4120-4122.
19. Korytnyk, W.; Valentekovic-Horvath; S, Petrie, C.R. Tetrahedron. 1982, 38, 2547-2550.
20. Isetin, B.; Reichstein, T. Helv. Chim. Acta. 1944, 27, 1146-1149.

21. Meindle, P.; Tuppy, H., Monatsh. Chem. 1969, 100, 1295-1306.
22. Gantt, R.; Millner, S.; Binkley, S.B. Biochemistry. 1964, 3, 1952-1960.
23. Shulman, M.L.; Khorlin, A. Ya. Carbohydr. Res. 1973, 27, 141-147.
24. Hough, L.; Penglis, A.E.; Richardson, A.C. Can. J. Chem. 1981, 59, 396-404.
25. Sharma, M.; Korytnyk, W. XIIIth. International Carbohydr. Symposium. 1986, 93.
26. Sharma, M.; Korytnyk, W. Carbohydr. Res. 1980, 79, 39-51.
27. Korytnyk, W.; Sharma, M.; Angelino, N.; Bernacki, R.J. XIIth International Carbohydr. Symposium. 1982, IV 40.
28. Garegg, P.J., Hultberg, H. Carbohydr. Res. 1981, 93, C10-C11.
29. Jaquinet, J.C.; Petil, J.M.; Sinay, P. Carbohydr. Res. 1974, 38, 305-311.
30. Burnett, J.E.G. Ciba Fdn. Symp. Elsevier and Associated Scientific Publishers, Amsterdam, 1972, 95-175.
31. Taylor, N.F. Ciba Fdn. Symp. Elsevier and Associated Scientific Publishers, Amsterdam, 1972, 215-238.
32. Niedbala, M.J.; Madiyalakin, R.; Matta, K., Crickard, K.; Sharma, M; and Bernacki, R.J. Cancer Res. 1987, 47, 4634-4641.
33. Bernacki, R.J.; Porter, C.W.; Korytnyk, W. and Mihich, E. Adv. Enzyme Regulat. 1977, 16, 217-237.
34. Morin, M.J.; Porter, C.W.; Petrie III, C.R.; Korytnyk, W. and Bernacki, R.J. Biochem. Pharmacol. 1973, 32, 553-561.
35. Sharma, R.A.; Kavai, I.; Fu, Y.L. and Bobek, M. Tetrahedron Lett. 1977, 39, 3433-3436.

RECEIVED January 18, 1988

Author Index

Affiliation Index

Subject Index

207

Production by Barbara J. Libengood
Indexing by Deborah H. Steiner and Linda R. Ross
Jacket design by Carla L. Clemens

Elements typeset by Hot Type Ltd., Washington, DC
Printed and bound by Maple Press, York, PA

Recent ACS Books

Biotechnology and Materials Science: Chemistry for the Future
Edited by Mary L. Good
160 pp; clothbound; ISBN 0–8412–1472–7

Chemical Demonstrations: A Sourcebook for Teachers
By Lee R. Summerlin and James L. Ealy, Jr.
Volume 1, Second Edition, 192 pp; spiral bound; ISBN 0–8412–1481–6

Chemical Demonstrations: A Sourcebook for Teachers
By Lee R. Summerlin, Christie L. Borgford, and Julie B. Ealy
Volume 2, Second Edition, 229 pp; spiral bound; ISBN 0–8412–1535–9

Practical Statistics for the Physical Sciences
By Larry L. Havlicek
ACS Professional Reference Book; 198 pp; clothbound; ISBN 0–8412–1453–0

The Basics of Technical Communicating
By B. Edward Cain
ACS Professional Reference Book; 198 pp; clothbound; ISBN 0–8412–1451–4

The ACS Style Guide: A Manual for Authors and Editors
Edited by Janet S. Dodd
264 pp; clothbound; ISBN 0–8412–0917–0

Personal Computers for Scientists: A Byte at a Time
By Glenn I. Ouchi
276 pp; clothbound; ISBN 0–8412–1000–4

Writing the Laboratory Notebook
By Howard M. Kanare
146 pp; clothbound; ISBN 0–8412–0906–5

Principles of Environmental Sampling
Edited by Lawrence H. Keith
458 pp; clothbound; ISBN 0–8412–1173–6

Phosphorus Chemistry in Everyday Living
By Arthur D. F. Toy and Edward N. Walsh
362 pp; clothbound; ISBN 0–8412–1002–0

Chemistry and Crime: From Sherlock Holmes to Today's Courtroom
Edited by Samuel M. Gerber
135 pp; clothbound; ISBN 0–8412–0784–4

For further information and a free catalog of ACS books, contact:
American Chemical Society
Distribution Office, Department 225
1155 16th Street, NW, Washington, DC 20036
Telephone 800–227–5558